Health, Technology and Society

Medicine, health care, and the wider social meaning and management of health are undergoing major changes. In part this reflects developments in science and technology, which enable new forms of diagnosis, treatment and delivery of health care. It also reflects changes in the locus of care and the social management of health. Locating technical developments in wider socio-economic and political processes, each book in the series discusses and critiques recent developments in health technologies in specific areas, drawing on a range of analyses provided by the social sciences. Some have a more theoretical focus, some a more applied focus but all draw on recent research by the authors. The series also looks toward the medium term in anticipating the likely configurations of health in advanced industrial society and does so comparatively, through exploring the globalization and internationalization of health.

Erik Aarden

Producing Citizenship in Medical Research Collections

palgrave
macmillan

Erik Aarden
Department of Society, Knowledge and Politics
University of Klagenfurt
Klagenfurt, Austria

ISSN 2946-3386 ISSN 2946-3378 (electronic)
Health, Technology and Society
ISBN 978-981-95-1706-0 ISBN 978-981-95-1707-7 (eBook)
https://doi.org/10.1007/978-981-95-1707-7

Cigdem Simsek

This Palgrave Macmillan imprint is published by the registered company Springer Nature Singapore Pte Ltd.
The registered company address is: 152 Beach Road, #21-01/04 Gateway East, Singapore 189721, Singapore

Preface and Acknowledgements

This book has been more than a decade in the making, from the start of a fellowship that allowed me to do much of the research for it in the Spring of 2012 to handing in the manuscript in early 2025. While I make some final changes, a pronounced sceptic of many advances in medical science and technology has just been confirmed to lead the massive conglomerate of public health agencies in the United States. At the same time, political parties and movements that aim to rewrite the history of probably the major health event of our lifetime, the COVID-19 pandemic, are gaining strength the world over. Often, their appeal seems to consist in large part in their questioning of and opposition to governmental responses to the pandemic as well as scientific consensus on its severity and on appropriate preventive and curative measures. You would therefore be excused for thinking this is an odd time to finish a book that critically examines the idea that the production of medical knowledge is a public good. Surely, there can be little doubt that tests, vaccines and treatments for COVID-19, many of them developed at breakneck speed to confront a newly emerging disease, have saved numerous lives[1]? I readily acknowledge that it is beyond my area of expertise to cast doubt on such statements. At the same time, I think it is perhaps more necessary than ever to understand the normative commitments shaping how medical knowledge gets claimed to be a public good. I think this is the only way to understand public misgivings about science and technology in the context of the pandemic, while simultaneously countering lies and hostility towards experts that emerged over the course of the pandemic. This is (for obvious temporal reasons) not precisely why I started work on this book, but I consider a brief pandemic excursion illuminating for sketching what I think are the stakes in writing this.

Ever since the SARS-CoV-2 virus started spreading around the world in the first few months of 2020, it regularly generated new surprises—in terms of its biological behaviour and the disease it caused, but also with regard to its societal effects (da Silva Torres et al., 2022). For some observers, the COVID-19 pandemic formed a challenge for the biomedical sciences first and foremost, requiring the application of frontier approaches and technologies in (post)genomics and bioinformatics (Pennington, 2022). As the medical sciences relatively swiftly proceeded to sequence the virus, develop tests and produce a vaccine, any shortcomings in addressing the pandemic seemed to be due to the ineptitude of governments and scientific ignorance (Barrett & Yaffe, 2020). Yet this proved to be an overly simplistic view. From early on in the pandemic, social scientists countered this narrative by stressing how medical science is "less than half the story" (Dingwall et al., 2013, p. 167) of what was happening. A pandemic does not only involve the spread of a virus (which is in and of itself not only biological). It also entails how this spread and efforts to "bend the curve" of new infections relate to human behaviour, social and political organization, fears, efforts at explanation and intervention, as well as persistent and new social inequalities (Will & Bendelow, 2020; Pickersgill, 2020).

Particular narratives that formed around the pandemic involved intersecting views of disease biology and social order, associated with particular ways of knowing. Warwick Anderson (2021), for example, has argued that disease modelling became a central pandemic knowledge technique. The implication of how the pandemic was modelled, then, was that populations were framed as biological rather than social entities. Modelling was thereby also an effort to depoliticize the pandemic and pandemic responses. Yet if we understand 'the political' to revolve around the question how we want to live together,[2] politics forms a vital component of how to handle a pandemic—or health and disease more generally.

Writing in the first months of 2025, where the pandemic is largely fading from view and becoming a thing of the past for many,[3] it seems needless to say that efforts at depoliticization failed. Although the pandemic formed a global phenomenon that, in the eyes of many, took 'the same' biological form across national borders, responses within these borders were vastly different. Individual countries developed distinct responses to the arrival and spread of COVID-19, each interpreting the disease differently and seeking situated responses that set different priorities in balancing health, civil liberties and economic interests (Jasanoff et al., 2021). Differences in responses to COVID-19 stretched from national policy strategies to the development and use of particular technologies to understand, trace and manage the pandemic. These included technologies as diverse as tests, vaccines, facemasks and contact tracing apps. Focusing on the latter in a comparison between Austria and Norway, Ingrid Metzler and Heidrun Åm (2022) have shown how these technologies do far more than mapping who has been close to whom. Technologies have also been pivotal in defining good citizenship during the pandemic. In nationally distinct ways, contract tracing apps as well as other technologies generated particular answers to questions such as which data the state may collect about its citizens, under which circumstances and how citizens are expected to behave to contain the spread of a virus. Technologies thereby exercise particular forms of power. As such, they are not merely neutral tools, but become contested in the context of responding to a pandemic as a social and political as well as a medical problem.

The widespread failure to recognize the pandemic as a sociopolitical issue, and thus a terrain of contested norms, values and ideas of the good life has certainly been an important factor in the rise of resistance to pandemic measures and the emergence of alternative narratives regarding its origins, impacts and solutions. While policy measures informed by medical research largely prioritized the protection of life and population health, many of these measures were questioned in terms of their effects on civil liberties and established ways of living (Jasanoff, 2020). To be sure, many people favoured pandemic measures such as lockdowns and contact restrictions for good reason. They were largely convinced that such measures served a general purpose and would help in protecting the lives of those most vulnerable to this new and largely unknown disease.

Yet the denial of uncertainty and of the political character of all response measures caused many people to raise doubts about how the pandemic was handled—doubts that in turn were often framed as ignorant and hostile to science, reason and general well-being (Harambam, 2023). Scepticism around pandemic policies thereby resonate with how Brian Wynne (2007, p. 105) and others have long argued that "many public concerns *relate to* the science [...] but are not *scientific* issues". This does not mean that any claim about the pandemic is as good as any other. Yet it does imply that the stakes are more complex than how to prevent or cure a disease alone. Health is, and should be treated as the deeply social and cultural aspect of (collective) life that it is.

In the context of the COVID-pandemic, Jaron Harambam (2020) has argued that the simultaneously biological and social character of the pandemic and many of the issues it raises make it a quintessential issue for scholars in science and technology studies (STS) to respond to. Yet despite this urgency, in his view we have largely been absent from the public debate. More than 4 years later, after misgivings about how the pandemic was handled have given rise to (or have at least been part of the repertoire of) authoritarian and extreme right movements throughout the democratic world, this question is perhaps more urgent than ever. My own position is that I have been reluctant to join the choir of academic commentaries early in the pandemic. In part, I was uncomfortable with how some colleagues seemed too eager to treat this 'crisis' as the infamous opportunity it allegedly always is. I am also not sure that STS efforts to parse questions of knowledge and trust would have had much of a political effect. The rise of extremist political movements in large parts of Europe and North America has many origins and in most cases, these movements have little patience for academic disciplines that question presumptions of essential, natural differences, social inequalities and structures of authority. Nevertheless, I think the important questions the pandemic has raised should make us acutely aware of the continued importance of trying to understand how science and technology figure in the contemporary world. This can and should include continued interrogation of scientific claims of knowledge and authority, while also recognizing how our thinking may be co-opted. We need to find a balance between critique as a mode of analysis and the risks of being read in terms that are diametrically opposed to our own visions of a desirable future of freedom and solidarity, which I think many in STS aspire to. My hope is to make an ever so tiny contribution to such thinking and to such futures with this book.

This book is not about COVID-19. Most of the research I report on had been done before the pandemic, and although each of the case studies can in one way or another be tied to pandemic responses, I chose not to trace those threads. Yet, my argument is in part that tracing normative and political commitments inscribed in scientific projects under 'normal' circumstances, may help in getting a clearer view of the political dimensions of knowing whenever science and health become more evidently 'political' in extreme situations. My starting point in the first chapter is the observation that claims towards an (moral) obligation to participate in research are problematic, because this presumes science to be a kind of unassailable good. Such claims fail to consider the sociopolitical dimensions or ramifications of medical research efforts. In many ways, the presumptions underlying such claims are similar to what caused opposition and hostility during the pandemic. My argument, by contrast, is that we can only really see the social value of medical science if we ask which 'social' we speak of. I intend to answer this question in the context of scientific data and tissue collections, which I describe as infrastructures for the purpose of population-based medical research. I do not argue that I provide a recipe for better social responses to uncertainty in the next pandemic. I do think this analysis can help us think about what may be done and to be realistic about the potential of research and how to address shortcomings in science.

The COVID-19 pandemic brought many of the themes discussed in this book to the foreground of public consciousness. It also made us more aware than ever of the importance of personal connections and of collective efforts to solve problems. Although there is only one name on the cover of this book, I have benefited tremendously from comments, ideas and support from various collectives of which I had the pleasure to be part. These collectives included many more people than the ones I mention here by name. My apologies upfront to anyone I have forgotten—it says more about my memory than about your contributions to my research, thinking and writing.

The work on which this book is based was undertaken in two research projects and positions at four institutions. Funding from the European Commission for a Marie Curie Outgoing Fellowship (project number PIOF-GA-2010-272996) and the Austrian Science Fund FWF for an international project (project number I 3982) enabled me to do research in a variety of different locations. As my institutional affiliations over the years, Maastricht University's Faculty of Arts and Social Sciences, the Harvard Program on Science, Technology and Society, the Department of Science and Technology Studies at the University of Vienna and the (now) Department of Society, Knowledge and Politics at the University of Klagenfurt provided solid grounding. Within the two projects, Sheila Jasanoff and Ulrike Felt both provided intellectual support and offered great insight. Wiebe Bijker not only supported me in applying for and carrying through with my Marie Curie fellowship, but generally opened up a whole new world as the person who first introduced me to STS as a student. His periodical words of advice and support throughout my academic career have been invaluable to getting me to a point I never thought I would ever be at.

Out of all the colleagues who participated in the research projects I have been involved in or who have supported me in other ways, there are some I would like to mention by name. It was a pleasure to work with Nina Klimburg-Witjes, Kamiel Mobach, Oguz Ozkan and Zinaida Vasilyeva in the METAFORIS project on European research infrastructures. Sebastian Pfotenhauer was one of the initiators of that project, a great collaborator in other work and a dear friend throughout the years. I have fond memories of time spent with many people in the Boston area, of whom I want to mention Za Barron, Alessandro Blasimme, Margo Boenig-Liptsin, Joakim Juhl, Luca Marelli, Zara Mirmalek and Daniela Schuh in particular. In Vienna, I was warmly welcomed to the department by and/or had many fruitful interactions with, among others, Kaya Akyüz, Dorothea Born, Kay Felder, Maximilian Fochler, Florentine Frantz, Melanie Goisauf, Susanne Öchsner Michael Penkler, Anna Pichelstorfer, Pouya Sepehr, Lisa Sigl and Paul Trauttmansdorff. I tried out many ideas in this book (and many more that didn't make it) on several cohorts of students in the Science-Technology-Society Master's programme in Vienna—who unknowingly have helped me refine my thinking. In Klagenfurt, I have found the time to finish this work while embarking in new directions—not least due to many enjoyable and supportive interactions with Daniel Barben, Anja Bauer, Christof Lammer, Julia Malik, Victoria Meklin and Helene Sorgner.

For longer than I think either of us cares to acknowledge, I have had a great sounding board and person to think with in Ingrid Metzler. I feel I learn something from every conversation we have and am delighted to be able to work on a joint project (that is, superficially, about the pandemic) as I am wrapping up work on this book.

I take infrastructure as one of the central concepts in my book. Since the invisibility of work is a key insight from infrastructure studies, I would also like to express my gratitude to the anonymous reviewers of various journals that have shared their thoughts on more and (not so rarely) less convincing versions of my manuscripts. Although I do not know who you are, you have made my writing and analysis better, often pointing me in directions I had not seen before. While review work is mostly unaccounted for, I hope this little token of appreciation gets seen by whomever it may concern.

Material presented in the following chapters has, in different forms, been published as "Repositioning Biological Citizenship: State, Population and Individual Risk in the Framingham Heart Study", *Biosocieties*. 13(2), 494–512 (Chap. 2); "Projecting and Producing 'Usefulness' of Biomedical Research Infrastructures; Or Why the Singapore Tissue Network Closed", *Science and Public Policy*, 44(6), 753–762; "'Samples Are Precious': Value Formations in the Potentiality and Practices of Biobanking in Singapore", *Science, Technology & Human Values*, 49(3), 500–523 (Chap. 3); "Decoding the Million Death Study: Ambivalence of Producing Evidence on Mortality in India", *Economic and Political Weekly*, 54(50), 41–48; "Human Sensing Infrastructures and Global Public Health Security in India's Million Death Study", in Nina Klimburg-Witjes, Nikolaus Pöchacker and Geoffrey Bowker (Eds.), *Sensing Security. Sensors as Transnational Security Infrastructures*, Manchester: Mattering Press, 136–162; "Ignorance and the Paradoxes of Evidence-Based Global Health: The Case of Mortality Statistics in India's Million Death Study", *Science as Culture*, 31(4), 433–454 (Chap. 4); "Infrastructuring European Scientific Integration: Heterogeneous

Meanings of the European Biobanking Infrastructure BBMRI-ERIC", *Social Studies of Science,* 53(4), 572–598; "Mapping Materials, Drawing Europe: Sample and Data Quality and Accessibility in the Biobanking Infrastructure BBMRI-ERIC", *Big Data & Society*, 12(1), 1–13 (Chap. 5); and "Making Value(s) Through Social Contracts for Biomedical Population Research", in Vincenzo Pavone and Joanne Goven (Eds), *Bioeconomies: Life, Technology and Capital in the 21st Century*, Basingstoke; Palgrave Macmillan, pp. 161–184.

All the people responding to presentations on parts of this work at academic meetings large and small have helped me forward as well. Indirectly, many of their suggestions and critiques have found their way into these pages. Interview respondents shall for the most part remain equally anonymous, but I am deeply indebted to their generosity in time and insight. While doing research in Singapore and India in particular, Mike Fischer, Catelijne Coopmans and the people of Tembusu College at the National University of Singapore as well as Ashawari Chaudhury, Poonam Pandey and Ambuj Sagar have provided invaluable support.

Many people at Palgrave Macmillan have made the publication of this book possible. While most of them remain invisible to me as well, I would in particular like to thank Rachael Ballard for first reaching out and showing interest in my idea and to Marion Duval for her patience in waiting for the manuscript and in answering this confused first-time author's many questions. Here, too, anonymous reviewers provided helpful feedback on the proposal and the manuscript.

My final thanks go to the people who have little to do with this book professionally, but have been and are all the more important for all else in life. Michaela Schmidt supports me in too many ways to count, but perhaps most importantly by taking my mind off of work. Unfortunately, I do not see my brothers Dirk and René, and their small and slightly larger families nearly enough, but the time we do have together means the world to me. Lastly, I want to dedicate this book to my parents and thank them for nothing less than everything.

Competing Interests The author has no competing interests to declare that are relevant to the content of this manuscript.

Notes

1. To give just one example, a modelling study of the effect of the first year of vaccination calculates that tens of millions of lives have been saved (Watson et al., 2022).
2. Moreover, in the context of COVID-19 and beyond, the question of living together also requires urgent attention to the way humans live with non-humans and its profound implications for health (Celermajer & McKibbin, 2023). This is a theme I will sideline in this book, although I do believe our relation to other species and the planet as a whole is probably our most pressing political concern going forward.
3. But by no means all, as the still largely unresolved puzzle of long COVID should remind us (Greenhalgh et al., 2024).

Series Editors' Preface

Medicine, health care and the wider social meanings and management of health are continually in the process of change. While the 'birth of the clinic' heralded the process through which health and illness became increasingly subject to the surveillance of medicine, for example, surveillance has become more complex, sophisticated and targeted—as seen in the search for 'precision medicine' and now 'precision public health'. Both surveillance and health itself emerge as more provisional, uncertain and risk-laden as a consequence, and we might also ask what now constitutes 'the clinic', how meaningful a concept of a clinic ultimately is, and where else might we now find (or not find) healthcare spaces and interventions.

Ongoing developments in science and technology are helping to enable and propel new forms of diagnosis, treatment and the delivery of health care. In many contexts, these innovations both reflect and further contribute to changes in the locus of care and burden of responsibility for health. Genetics, informatics, imaging—to name but a few—are redefining collective and individual understandings of the body, health and disease. At the same time, long established and even ostensibly mundane technologies and techniques can generate ripples in local discourse and practices as ideas about the nature and focus of healthcare shift in response to global debates about, for instance, One Health and Planetary Health.

The very technologies that (re)define health are also the means through which the individualization of health care can occur—through, for instance, digital health, diagnostic tests and the commodification of restorative tissue. This individualization of health is both culturally-derived and state-sponsored, as exemplified by the promotion of 'self-care'. These shifts are simultaneously welcomed and contested by professionals, patients and wider publics. Hence they at once signal and instantiate wider societal ambivalences and divisions.

This Series explores these processes within and beyond the conventional domain of 'the clinic', and asks whether they amount to a qualitative shift in the social ordering and value of medicine and health. Locating technical use and developments in wider socio-economic and political processes, each book discusses and critiques the dynamics between health, technology and society through a variety of specific cases, and drawing on a range of analyses provided by the social sciences.

The Series has already published more than 30 books that have explored many of these issues, drawing on novel, critical and deeply informed research undertaken by their authors. In doing so, the books have shown how the boundaries between the three core dimensions that underpin the whole Series—health, technology and society—are changing in fundamental ways.

Erik Aarden's monograph, *Producing Citizenship in Medical Research Collections*, explores the imbricating social and epistemic dimensions of population studies across countries and continents. Based on careful, rigorously conducted interviews and documentary analysis, Aarden addresses not only questions about the role of infrastructures in constituting knowledge and populations, but also about ontologies of disease, about bio-economies and about the role of 'big data' in science and societies. Through nuanced and engagingly presented analysis, Aarden demonstrates that different instantiations of population health research synthesize distinct conceptions of citizenship, with ensuing implications for participant and community rights and responsibilities. This highly original and important study invites fresh attention to the politics and practices of population health in evermore global(ized) contexts.

London, UK
Edinburgh, UK

Rebecca Lynch
Martyn Pickersgill

Contents

Abbreviations

A*STAR	Agency for Science, Technology and Research (Singapore)
AI	Artificial Intelligence
BAC	Bioethics Advisory Commission (Singapore)
BBMRI-ERIC	Biobanking and BioMolecular Resources Research Infrastructure–European Research Infrastructure Consortium
BMSI	Biomedical Sciences Initiative (Singapore)
BU	Boston University (United States)
CME	Central Medical Evaluation (Million Death Study)
CVD	Cardiovascular disease
dbGaP	Database of Genotypes and Phenotypes (United States)
DG	Director General
DNA	Deoxyribonucleic acid
EATRIS	European Infrastructure for Translational Medicine
ELSI	Ethical, Legal and Social Issues
ERIC	European Research Infrastructure Consortium (European Union)
ESFRI	European Strategy Forum on Research Infrastructures (European Union)
EU	European Union
FHS	Framingham Heart Study
GDP	Gross Domestic Product
GWAS	Genome-Wide Association Studies

HGP	Human Genome Project
ICD-10	International Classification of Diseases, Tenth Edition
ISBER	International Society for Biological and Environmental Repositories
IT	Information Technology
JAMA	Journal of the American Medical Association
MDS	Million Death Study
NHLBI	National Heart, Lung and Blood Institute (United States)
NIH	National Institutes of Health (United States)
RGI	Office of the Registrar General of India
SBB	Singapore BioBank
SRS	Sample Registration System (India)
STN	Singapore Tissue Network
STS	Science and Technology Studies
US	United States
VA	Verbal Autopsy

List of Figures

List of Tables

1

Introducing Medical Research Collections as Sources of 'Public Goods'?

Do people have a (moral) obligation to participate in medical research? This question was raised, and answered in the affirmative, by three US based medical researchers in a 2009 paper in the *Journal of the American Medical Associations* (JAMA). According to these authors (Owen Schaefer et al., 2009), the very fact that medical research produces a collectively available good in the form of generalizable medical knowledge implies that any of us, if we want to benefit from such knowledge in the context of health care in the future, should make our small but significant contribution to producing knowledge in the present. Even though the authors acknowledge that there are hurdles that make some of this knowledge (and its technical application in new diagnostics and therapies) more easily or quickly accessible to some than to others, they see this as a problem of pragmatics rather than principle. Medical knowledge, they imply, will "trickle down" and thus be a benefit—and hence responsibility—for us all.

Following a similar line of argumentation, an article in *The New York Times* in April 2017 made the plea that "science needs your cells" (Fernandez Lynch & Joffe, 2017). The authors Holly Fernandez Lynch and Steven Joffe, both health policy and ethics academics at prestigious US universities at the time, dug back to the by now famous story of Henrietta Lacks (which had just come out as a movie in 2017) to support

E. Aarden, *Producing Citizenship in Medical Research Collections*, Health, Technology and Society, https://doi.org/10.1007/978-981-95-1707-7_1

their argument. Among the injustices that characterize that particular story, they argued, the use of the cells as such is not one of them. Instead, the authors maintained that most restrictions on research use of cells—including asking for consent—would be "worrisome because its benefits are so great". However, Fernandez Lynch and Joffe are a bit more careful in their endorsement of such benefits as a straightforward collective good, pointing out the importance of privacy protections and arguing for a "push for universal health care to ensure that the benefits of the research are available to all".

On the other side of the spectrum, commentators hold against a moral obligation for research participation. The German cardiologist Christian Seiler (2018), for example, sees research participation in a potential tension with clinical ethics. He argued that to see a refusal to participate as immoral would contradict the individual autonomy of the patient and complicate the relationship of trust with their treating physician. This perspective implies that an obligation to participate might create additional obstacles to benefit from medical knowledge at the individual level. Moreover, as the aforementioned plea for universal health care suggests, the idea of knowledge as a public good requires a number of assumptions about the benefits of research and how they get distributed (Rennie, 2011). Health care access is just one among several potential issues in this regard. Others include the idea that medical research is not only (by definition) beneficial to all, but also the best possible way to address problems of ill health. Yet this position requires, at the very least, ignoring selective priority-setting in research as well as the various non-medical determinants of health. Moreover, the idea of a moral obligation can imply a disempowerment of research participants if the default position is that they should participate. This is particularly problematic in light of existing inequalities, where "the lion's share of research benefits [...] tend to flow to those already better off" (Rennie, 2011, p. 45), only arriving much later to the poor and marginalized—if ever. Thus, the idea of a moral obligation to participate in research appears to ignore important aspects of both how medical knowledge gets produced and how and to whom its outputs actually become available.

The question if and when individuals have an obligation to participate in medical research is also discussed in domains such as the use of medical data (Seidenberg, 2014) and medical artificial intelligence (AI) (Müller, 2022). What these domains have in common is that a professed need for *large collections of data and tissue* are at the centre of the debate. Building large collections quite obviously requires a lot of people to participate or donate data and tissue. But it is not straightforward to presume that all of these people *should* donate, because they *stand to benefit* from the research done with the collected materials (Knoppers, 2005). To be able to assess whether this claim has any merit, we should therefore look at whether the claim that medical knowledge is a good available to all bears out in practice. This requires looking at how medical research collections frame both medical knowledge and the collective of (future) patients whom it addresses. This is the aim of this book, in which I trace how specific notions of health and disease and specific human collectives become what Bruno Latour (2004) might have described as "matters of concern" in medical research. More specifically, I look in detail at four publicly funded efforts to collect and store human tissue materials and/or data that serve as *infrastructures for the purpose of population-based medical research.* These infrastructures have been established at different points in time and for different purposes in different parts of the world—ranging from a decades old study of heart disease risks in the United States to a short-lived initiative to centralize the storage of tissue collected for research in Singapore, and from an ongoing study of the causal distribution of mortality in India to a Europe-wide network for facilitating exchange of stored materials and data.

My central aims in considering these four cases in parallel to each other are threefold. First, I aim to contrast different situated medical collection initiatives to explore how medical knowledge and its publics get coproduced (Jasanoff, 2004) under distinct circumstances. At the same time, I also look for similarities between the cases to answer the broader question if and how conceptions of medical knowledge as a public good are articulated or contradicted across a range of distinct medical research efforts. Finally, I use these four cases to develop an analytical heuristic for interrogating how infrastructures for the purpose of population-based medical research generate a set of rights and responsibilities (that I will conceptualize in terms of citizenship) for not only research participants, but wider (national) populations—and beyond—as well.

In the remainder of this chapter, I will map out the broader landscape through which this book travels. I first consider how, especially since the completion of the Human Genome Project (HGP), arguments around the growing scale of medical research (which are not limited to the field of genomics, as I will show) are tied up with promises about the benefits of research. Research in the social sciences and humanities has shown how such promises—especially in the context of data and tissue collections—shape research agendas, but also raise questions about the meaning of 'big' in the alleged emergence of big biology. By interrogating the focus on size this notion suggests, I will move to a broader discussion of how organization and practices of medical sciences relate and suggest that the notion of infrastructure is useful to capture the various dimensions of this issue. I then move to the question of ethics in relation to large research collections (commonly labelled 'biobanks') before suggesting that a register of justice is more fitting to explore if and how promises of progress come to fruition in medical research collections. Based on these strands of literature, I suggest that the conceptualization of research collections as infrastructures for the purpose of population-based medical research and a detailed exploration of such infrastructures' inner mechanics of governance and knowledge production can provide insight into how specific 'goods' for specific 'publics' get constructed. I will therefore end the chapter with a brief description of my approach to the four case studies, before introducing the cases in more detail and sketching out the argument that follows.

Promises in 'Big' Medical Research Collections

Central to the argument for a moral obligation to participate in medical research is the idea that increasingly large numbers of research participants are required to answer the most pressing current research questions. Large scale research and sharing of data are considered essential not only in genomics research (Stark et al., 2025), but also in, for example, the medical use of artificial intelligence (Akyüz et al., 2024). Large collections of human tissue and—above all—medical data are supposed to enable the identification of how minute biological differences between people affect the development of disease. The argument for so-called 'big biology' is hence related to the recognition that increased insight into the human genome has laid bare the complexity of disease biology (Check Hayden, 2010). Associated with this is a shift in medicine from identifying genetic mutations that are strongly predictive of disease to changes in the genome that either correspond to only slightly increased risks or are only consequential in relation to other factors. Likewise, recent claims that AI can help diagnose, for example, skin cancer more quickly and accurately than human doctors rely on the training of algorithms that recognize patterns in large sets of cancer images (Beltrami et al., 2022). Since large datasets of unique cases—not to mention control groups of unaffected people—require contributions from many people both healthy and ill, increasing participation in medical research is considered of great importance here as well.

The desire for larger datasets and growing numbers of research participants is part of what some commentators see as a trend towards big biology. This notion further implies growing numbers of people and institutions involved in any one research project or consortium as well as rising amounts of funding (Vermeulen et al., 2013). This trend is further associated with particular normative assumptions regarding future directions in life science research. Claims around big biology entail "normative assumptions that bigger will be faster, and that faster will be better" (Davies et al., 2013, p. 387), producing, among other things, new diagnostics and therapeutics in a shorter timeframe. Assumptions like this are reflected in the scale of research practices, management and discourses.

Key aspects of big biology in the context of human health research crystallize in (networks of) repositories of human tissue and data, which are often described as "biobanks" (Lieb et al., 2024)[1]. One influential definition describes them as "structured collections of biological samples and associated data stored for the purposes of present and future research" (Parodi, 2015, p. 15). Such repositories have a (fairly) long history in medical science going back to, for example, materials stored from newborn screening or tumour tissue being kept in hospital storage.[2] Yet, the idea of collecting body materials and health data from large cohorts took on additional prominence in medical research after the completion of the Human Genome Project. A key aspect of such 'new' biobanks (which nevertheless built on existing collections) was the promise to enable research on the interactions between genes, lifestyle and environment as causal factors for disease (Davis & Khoury, 2007). Based on such promises of improving population health, but also of developing new, marketable technologies, (national) biobanks were established in many places around the world in the first decade of this century (Kaiser, 2002; Trivedi, 2008).

In line with the idea that they would enable research on the genomic dimensions of common diseases, biobank projects have been described as "a gold mine for improving health care" (Kaiser, 2002, p. 1160). Furthermore, efforts to connect and harmonize biobanks into larger, potentially global networks were—organizational and ethical complexities notwithstanding—expected to increase the potential of research even further (Knoppers et al., 2007; Shickle & Griffin, 2009; Hewitt & Hainaut, 2011). Biobanking has therefore been described as an "infrastructure science" (Knoppers & Hudson, 2011, p. 329), laying the groundwork, as it were, for new areas of medical research more equipped for understanding the complexities of human health and disease.

This image of large amounts of materials and data contributing to better research and more solid evidence on what causes disease is not unique to high-tech domains in (post)genomic research and artificial intelligence. The question of large numbers and the (big) scale of research is also increasingly important in the domain of global health. In this context, it may be argued that the use of quantitative metrics and ideas of solutions transferable across scale are what distinguishes global from international health (Birn, 2009; Adams, 2016; Gaudillière & Gasnier, 2020). Noteworthy about global health is further how the use of increasingly 'big' data is also tied in with a growing scale of actors and institutions that include both North-South academic partnerships (Crane, 2010) and so-called philantrocapitalist organizations (Global Health Watch, 2011; McGoey, 2015). The growing importance of quantitative metrics for developing and evaluating health interventions thereby suggests a "trust in numbers" (Porter, 1996) that is not altogether too different from the call for large numbers of participants in genomic biobanks. While the motivations for and forms of quantification in global health may thus be different, the similarities across domains of research suggest that there is a wider trend towards scaling up in medical research, which has particular implications for how the public good of research gets pursued and perceived (Pfotenhauer et al., 2022).

Various anthropological studies have reconstructed the meaning of metrics and quantification in global health 'on the ground' to question what numbers do and do not capture. They have shown, for example, how reliance on numbers forms not only a specific form of evidence, but also aligns with a specific politics of health on a global scale (Adams, 2016). Such research has further shown the selective and situationally specific production of numbers (Biruk, 2012). Quantification thereby often ignores local specificities and generates particular framings of health and disease that allow the circulation of research methods and findings between locations (Biehl & Petryna, 2013).

While such analyses question how the large scale of medical research comes into being, they simultaneously point to the power of persuasion size seems to possess. The power of arguments for scale in medical research reflect broader social expectations, promises and imaginations attributed to 'big biology', or the "potentiality" attributed to medical research and innovation (Taussig et al., 2013). This notion points to how benefits and futures imagined for biomedical research are reflected in the material manifestations of science while simultaneously producing moral imperatives for research.

For national biobanks established around the conclusion of the Human Genome Project with the explicit aim to gather materials from a representative sample of a given population, potentiality often includes an amalgam of social, political and cultural aims (Tutton, 2010). One particularly significant example is the UK Biobank, which was established in the early 2000s. In this initiative, different expectations of biobanking's value were interwoven with imaginaries of British strengths. A rhetoric of unique national characteristics such as the low threshold for medical care in the tax-funded National Health Service and the ethnic diversity of the population were tied together with notions of solidarity and innovation to argue for the biobank's value (Busby & Martin, 2006). Providing similar observations, Ruha Benjamin (2009) has described how postcolonial national genome projects pursued an idea of genomic sovereignty in response to political and commercial reconfigurations of the life sciences in the early twenty-first century. Countries pursuing "a lab of their own" do not only do so out of scientific interest, but also in an effort to reap the anticipated benefits of economic growth as well as global political and cultural significance from medical research.

Promises and expectations of future progress in "health and wealth" in medical research (Gardner & Webster, 2016) are central to many biobanking projects and the field of genomics at large (Tupasela, 2006; Martin, 2018). Mary-Jo DelVecchio-Good (2007, p. 377) refers to how the "biotechnical embrace" of contemporary high-tech medicine creates "a popular culture that is enamored with the biology of hope", an observation that suits the expectations around genomic biobanks. Discussing another high profile example, Mike Fortun (2008, p. 10) attends to the importance of hope in relation to the Icelandic Health Sector Database and maps out how promise is "an irreducible feature of genomics". He describes the Human Genome Project as a "fantastic infrastructure" in which visions and dreams get meshed together with mundane tools to produce an industry centred on promises rather than products. These promises travel to Iceland where they are part of a vision of a promising future, while simultaneously helping to create it. Similar to other cases of (national) biobanks, this future was weaving together scientific proficiency, commercial potential and national identity (Winickoff, 2006). Yet, Fortun also shows how activists questioning the ethical and commercial commitments of the Health Sector Database were able to show cracks in the discourse of promise. He thereby makes clear how promises are not only constitutive of the life sciences today, but may also give rise to critical assessment of claims regarding the public benefits of research.

Expectations of (future) value are also key in shaping discourses of commercial potential and speculation around the life sciences and biobanks (Turner et al., 2013). The economics of medical research and its potential productivity are a contested topic in social science analyses around concepts such as biocapital, biovalue and knowledge assets (Sunder Rajan, 2006; Cooper, 2008; Birch & Tyfield, 2013; Chiapetta & Birch, 2018). But these various perspectives largely agree that promises of future monetary gains from research form an important driver of many research initiatives. Research practices, organization and funding of research are in part shaped by, but also influence, how tissue collections, datasets and knowledge claims are valued. Yet the attribution of value to materials, data, knowledge—or even populations as a whole (Tarkkala & Tupasela, 2018)—should not exclusively be sought in 'the market'. Multiple studies of postgenomic life sciences have shown how various forms of value may be attributed to materials, data, as well as scientific work (Ankeny & Leonelli, 2015; Pinel et al., 2020; Pinel, 2021). Value in the life sciences is not exclusively economic, nor is it given in advance. Rather, different forms of value may be pursued and produced in distinct domains of biomedical research and health care—including in biobanking—and it depends on wider sociopolitical priorities and relations which kinds of value will be prioritized in particular cases (Tupasela, 2006; Burton et al., 2021).

To sum up, expected benefits to arise from medical research may be found in different places. Expectations of future value are associated with the mere existence of material and institutional formations for research, such as biobanks. A range of social science research has shown how biobanking projects are rooted in a belief that they have value in and of themselves. They promise to generate scientific proficiency, social cohesion, economic progress and various other advancements without wasting much effort on explaining how these benefits will germinate. As Sebastian Pfotenhauer, Joakim Juhl and myself (2019) have observed, this idea that scientific or technological innovation is both a necessary and sufficient response to a host of social problems is widespread in contemporary politics and public discourse. Surely, this "innovation imperative" is also deeply ingrained in today's medical research landscape, where it is often framed in terms of 'translation' between the scientific laboratory 'bench' and the applied clinical and/or commercial 'bedside' (Woolf, 2008; Levin & Danesh-Meyer, 2010; Collins, 2011; Cohrs et al., 2015).

However, the value attributed to or anticipated from stored materials and data as well as from the work done with those materials is considered to be more elusive. This, one might argue, is the key issue in translational medicine, which has itself advanced to become a discipline in medical research. Various observers have noted how the medical innovation 'pipeline' is neither unidirectional, nor is it particularly straight (Jogalekar, 2012; Vignola-Gagne & Biegelbauer, 2013; Van der Laan & Boenink,

2015). Clinical translation may be read as a promise that research generates collective benefits, but it is also described as a treacherous road, filled with many heterogeneous obstacles that require tailored interventions (Butler, 2008; Meslin et al., 2013). Translation has consequently been framed differently in different places, in line with specific political and cultural imaginations and expectations of how science and innovation contribute to better health care, economic advancement and other forms of social progress (Blümel, 2018; Aarden et al., 2021). Seeing clinical translation as a culturally situated phenomenon in relation to specific material and institutional formations for research then raises the question how research efforts intersect with efforts to generate societal benefits. Clinical translation thereby forms but one instance of the kinds of promises associated with medical research, but is particularly illustrative for how research practice and research governance intersect.

Practices and Governance of 'Big' Medical Research

While the rhetoric around recent trends in medical research and science policy suggests that research is growing bigger, philosophers, historians and other analysts of contemporary science have suggested that size may not be the distinctive element in how the life sciences are transforming. For example, Bruno Strasser (2012) has suggested in his analysis of the significance of 'big data' for the life sciences that the idea that overwhelming amounts of data pose a major challenge to scientists is not new. This claim ignores previous periodical outcries of concern that biologists generated more data than they could handle. Strasser therefore maintains that it is not the amount of data per se, but the shift from the field to the laboratory—and associated separation of data collection and analysis—that has changed the character of research in the life sciences. Moreover, it is questionable whether growing amounts of data as such are really the key to present transformations in biological research.

Despite such critiques focused on 'big biology' as a form of big data science, the growing importance of data is a key aspect of contemporary biology. In her book *Data-Centric Biology: A Philosophical Study*, Sabina Leonelli (2016) explores what data in science is, how it figures in biological research and with what effects for knowledge production. She argues that the focus on data has given rise to new data handling and dissemination practices that are shaped by new technologies and regulations for the production, storage, circulation, use and other practices related to data. These, in turn, have given rise to new kinds of institutions and professions in science (Ankeny & Leonelli, 2015). Central to the new importance of data in biology is, furthermore, its ability to travel between locations (Bates et al., 2016; Leonelli, 2020). This is not self-evident. It requires forms of preparation and packaging that make data fit to travel, but also involves imaginations of such travels and of possible destinations already in the production of data (Metzler et al., 2023). Data is shaped and imagined in relation to particular material and institutional conditions that, in turn, render data situational and relational. Data does not have essential characteristics, but changes form and meaning as it travels (Leonelli, 2016). This raises questions about the particular significance—or value—of data under specific circumstances (Fiske et al., 2022). Taking the notion that data is central to contemporary biological research seriously, then, raises the question how data practices feature into the alleged production of public goods in science.

The answer to this question is twofold, as it concerns both scientific practice and governance. These dimensions cannot neatly be separated, yet I will do so momentarily to sketch out different aspects of the question. Within science and technology studies (STS), the study of the production and evaluation of knowledge claims in practice has formed a foundational strand of research. So-called laboratory studies have attended to both the material and social configurations of knowledge making in (primarily) natural science laboratories as sites of scientific work *par excellence* (Pickering, 1992; Sismondo, 2009). As Karin Knorr Cetina (1983) has observed in an early review of such work, laboratory studies mostly entail ethnographic research on how science gets done, research objects get made and knowledge gets produced in laboratories. A main theme in laboratory studies, then, has been to show how knowledge is contingent on practices (but see (Doing, 2008) for a critique). In laboratories, researchers produce knowledge objects that are material, selective, contingent and socially situated. While material conditions shape what can and cannot be done in a laboratory, knowledge objects are equally conditioned by and situated in social relations both within and beyond the lab. In terms of the high expectations related to tissue and data collections in medical research, this approach invites several questions concerning practices and governance of research.

One of these questions concerns the making of research objects and their relations to knowledge about the world. Focusing on synthesization of proteins, Hans-Jörg Rheinberger (1997) has described the making and circulation of objects he describes as "epistemic things". In his study, he positioned epistemic things as components of experimental systems built at the interface of what is currently known and what is not. Experimental systems are hybrid settings that incorporate "the genuine working units of contemporary science in which scientific objects and the technical conditions of their production are inextricably interconnected" (Rheinberger, 1997, p. 2). In other words, to know an object requires making that object at the same time. Epistemic things are thereby not mere objects but are "things embodying concepts" (Rheinberger, 1997, p. 3). This notion thereby emphasizes how the creation of knowledge objects is located in space and time and shaped by both material and theoretical considerations that jointly generate representations, or models, of an object. The particular way knowledge objects are represented thereby account for the credibility of modern science.

Other perspectives in the study of scientific laboratories go into detail in describing the reconfiguration of natural phenomena into a form accessible to laboratory bench work (Knorr-Cetina, 1999). Among the most influential of these studies, Bruno Latour and Steve Woolgar's (1986) *Laboratory Life: The Construction of Scientific Facts* has introduced several key concepts in STS. Latour and Woolgar (1986, p. 32) propose a symmetrical treatment of social and material aspects of scientific knowledge production to trace the "process through which scientists give meaning to observations" and "how scientific order is constructed out of chaos" (Latour & Woolgar, 1986, p. 33). Central to this endeavour is their metaphor of "literary inscription" (Latour & Woolgar, 1986, p. 45) and reference to laboratory technologies as "inscription devices" that "transform pieces of matter into written documents" (Latour & Woolgar, 1986,

p. 54). They see credible knowledge claims as the outcome of building and extending a network of interrelated inscriptions and references (see also Latour, 1987, 1999). Claims building on inscriptions produced by devices ranging from laboratory machineries to texts, tables and figures subsequently become certified by obscuring the process of knowledge production and presenting the fact as the cause of its experimental proof rather than the other way around.

Knowledge claims not only gain credibility within the laboratory or even scientific community at large. As Latour (1983) has argued on the basis of Pasteur's work with microbes, the credibility of scientific claims is produced together with the formulation of social actors' interests. Central to Pasteur's success was his ability to "enrol" relevant social actors in his network and make them believe their interests aligned with Pasteur's knowledge claims. As Latour (1983, p. 167) writes "[t]here is no outside of science but there are long, narrow networks that make possible the circulation of scientific facts". These networks extend outside the lab and include practitioners (e.g., farmers in Pasteur's case), government agencies, professional organizations, but also the material, non-human elements involved. Latour argues that the laboratory is extended into the outside world and that its practices (re)shape social and natural relations. For Latour, the credibility of knowledge claims thereby roots in the making of heterogeneous networks that include but extend beyond laboratories.

In response to the tradition of laboratory studies, however, Thomas Gieryn (1995, p. 405), points out how studies of scientific practice cannot account for the 'cultural authority of science' beyond the credibility of specific knowledge claims. Gieryn (1999) therefore proposes an approach to scientific authority that develops a "cultural cartography" of science, focused on the "boundary work" of defining and demarcating science from other cultural domains in public representations. He argues that science is "[n]othing but a *space*, one that acquires its authority precisely from and through episodic negotiations of its flexible and contextually contingent borders and territories" (Gieryn 1995, p. 405). Although the characteristics of this space are "not so elastic that they may stretch endlessly in any direction" (Gieryn, 1999, p. 21), it is contextually specific what 'science' comes to mean. This meaning, moreover, is not only determined by scientists building networks alone, but also in a range of other institutions that regulate, fund, use and ask for scientific research.

Returning to the life sciences and the idea of 'big biology' in particular, Steven Hilgartner (2017) has described the intersections of scientific practice and the maintenance of public authority in the Human Genome Project with the concept of knowledge-control regimes. He develops this notion to attend to the governance of both knowledge production processes and of knowledge itself. He defines such regimes as "a sociotechnical arrangement that constitutes categories of agents, spaces, objects and relationships among them in a manner that allocates entitlements and burdens pertaining to knowledge" (Hilgartner, 2017, p. 9). Knowledge-control regimes thereby provide a "governing frame" (Hilgartner, 2017, p. 11) for scientific knowledge. These regimes changed and adapted along with the ways the HGP transformed both ways of doing and of organizing biological research. Thereby, "the epistemic problem of constructing knowledge and the sociopolitical one of constructing control over knowledge are tightly intertwined in the HGP" (Hilgartner, 2017, p. 89). With regard to contemporary biological and medical knowledge, Hilgartner thereby shows how scientific practice and governance intersect with each other.

Developing a similar argument with regard to the emergence of increasingly tight entanglements between research on normal and on pathological biological functions—in other words, biomedical research—Peter Keating and Alberto Cambrosio (2003) proposed the idea of biomedical platforms to make sense of institutional and regulatory configurations of contemporary science. They define platforms as "material and discursive arrangements that act at the bench upon which conventions concerning the biological or normal are connected with conventions concerning the medical or pathological" (Keating & Cambrosio, 2003, p. 4). They thereby also frame biomedical research as a sociotechnical construct in which practices of knowledge production, the governance of such practices and the governance of knowledge itself intermingle. In particular, they understand platforms to include a range of technoscientific, organizational, regulatory and other objects and discourses, arranged in such a way that they allow the circulation of things and ideas pertaining to health and disease.

In work that develops the idea of biomedical platforms further, Keating, Cambrosio and colleagues harken back to the idea of translation I introduced earlier to describe how biomedical objects get made and become meaningful in practice. They introduce the notion of regulatory objectivity (Cambrosio et al., 2006) to emphasize how regulatory requirements for the evaluation and market admission of new diagnostics and therapeutics has shaped criteria for evaluating biomedical knowledge claims. They thereby propose that other criteria than reference to some abstract truth shape the making of biomedical knowledge. Some notion of application, they suggest, is always already present, for example in the context of translational research. Both research and clinical application in the context of genomics are shaped in a "regime of actionability" that also involves consideration of regulatory preconditions for permitted clinical uses of knowledge as part of laboratory research (Keating et al., 2016). Genomic research thereby generates regulatory-scientific hybrids in efforts to understand and intervene in life (Kohli-Laven et al., 2011), shaping medicine to be what Catherine Waldby (2012) has described as an intersection of care and experiment in which both cannot be separated from dimensions of regulation and governance.

These various perspectives on the practices and governance of biological and biomedical research suggest that the conditions under which knowledge is produced are simultaneously socio-institutional and techno-epistemic, while also being tightly interwoven with the uses of this knowledge. Building on insights from the literature discussed above, I propose to develop the notion of *infrastructures for the purpose of population-based medical research* as a heuristic to further explore the intersections between knowledge (production) practices and governance in medical tissue and data collection efforts. While I untangle this heuristic further throughout this book, I centrally rely on the concept of infrastructure for its conceptual duality. On the one hand, infrastructure illuminates the (often invisible and neglected) sociomaterial work of creating the preconditions for other work (Star, 1999; Slota & Bowker, 2017). On the other hand, it also captures the (far more visible) promises and imaginaries of future progress often associated with infrastructure (Larkin, 2013; Anand et al., 2018). Furthermore, the kinds of promises and expectations associated with purposes of medical research and innovation can serve as infrastructure for how further research is pursued (Metzler, 2020). Infrastructure can thereby help explore why, and with which expectations of future benefit, medical science is organized and done in a particular way.

Against this background, it is worth noting how governance of science and technology—and, I would add, thereby the configuration of these infrastructures—may show significant differences across borders. Many comparative analyses in STS have shown how ostensibly 'the same' science (and technology) is interpreted, organized and regulated in significantly different ways from one jurisdiction to the next (Jasanoff, 2005; Parthasarathy, 2007, 2017; Aarden, 2016; Aarden et al., 2011). However, such analyses of cross-border differences in the organization and governance of science and its products raises some salient questions with regard to big biology and its emphasis on cross-border networks and growing scales of scientific work (see, e.g., Fischer, 2007). Although the comparative literature in STS mostly focuses on governance of science rather than research practices, legal and cultural cross-border differences are seen as a major challenge to international collaboration in biobanking (Kaye, 2009). In addition, differences in regulation and organization (Gottweis et al., 2009) and global political and economic asymmetries (Prasad, 2014b) do affect research practices. To consider such difference, it is therefore not only worthwhile to take a comparative approach to infrastructures for the purpose of population-based medical research, but to also consider how questions of ethics and justice figure into science.

Ethics and Justice in Medical Population Research Collections

The governance of medical research collections or biobanks, in particular, can take divergent forms across borders (Gille et al., 2020), in part due to the range of ethical issues they invoke. Several ethicists have pointed out how the ethics of biobanks are particular due to their large size, the limits of individual autonomy and the possible use of materials beyond the limits of individual consent (Rothstein, 2005; Knoppers & Abdul-Rahman, 2009).

One of the specific issues related to biobanks is their collective nature, which poses a challenge due to the primary orientation of ethical principles towards individual rights and interests (Mauron, 2008). This issue is related to the ethical issues raised by developments in molecular genetics since the 1990s (Fobelets & Nys, 2009). Individual notions of consent and confidentiality that have been at the core of medical research ethics are based on an individual vulnerability to harm and thereby ill-equipped for dealing with the collective nature of much genetic information (Widdows & Cordell, 2011). By its very nature, genetic information from any one individual always contains information about their biological relatives and (potentially) wider population groups as well. A key issue in medical research ethics related to genomics and biobanking has therefore been to develop new principles and approaches more tailored to these characteristics (Knoppers & Chadwick, 2005). This can, for example, be seen in discussions about a wide range of possible mechanisms of not only specific, but also 'broad' or 'blanket' consent. Such ideas not only seek to adjust protections for research participants to the genomic age, but also aim to facilitate long-term use of materials, regardless of the purposes for which they have initially been collected and stored (Otlowski, 2009; Sheehan, 2011; Mikkelsen et al., 2019; Smilan, 2022).

Within medical research, "biobank research and genomic information are reshaping our notions of health and medicine and offering the promise of more tailored medical treatment" (Mascalzoni, 2015, p. 1), thereby raising a range of questions with regard to how to govern biobanks. Various ethicists have pointed out that such governance can take a variety of forms—which is usually seen as an obstacle for harmonization (Chadwick & Strange, 2009)—yet emphasize a particular set of issues. Among the most prominent ethical concerns associated with biobanks in the literature are questions of donor privacy, (various forms of) consent and commercialization of biobank resources as well as sharing of its benefits (Knoppers & Abdul-Rahman, 2008; Kaye & Stranger, 2009; Widdows & Mullen, 2009; Tutton, 2010).

In light of the widespread discussion of whether and how biobanking benefits should be shared with donors, this literature often has little to say about what these benefits actually *are* (Pullman et al., 2012; Gottweis & Lauss, 2010). As Alan Petersen has observed, the ethics of biobanking is often framed narrowly, while "[t]he basic scientific premises underlying projects have been mostly unquestioned in the broader public domain" (Petersen, 2011, p. 56). Anne Kerr (2004, p. 117) concurred in describing ethics in biobanking as a "way in which discussions of the political economy of biobanks are sidelined in favour of the discourse of individual choice and progress in the fight against disease: two common tropes of late modernity". Kerr thereby draws attention to the problematic assumptions underlying the idea that ethical principles form a sufficient consideration of the normative implications and effects of population-scale biomedical research and how the promise of progress obscures more precise consideration of what biobanks are for. This is not to deny the value of medical research and of tissue and data collection and storage per se. Yet bringing political economy from the sideline onto the playing field enables a profound discussion of the consequences of how medical research gets organized and done. It thereby opens up a conversation about if and how individuals should participate that is obscured by references to a presumed public good somehow available to everyone.

Recent discussions around biobanking in Africa may illustrate how ethical issues intersect with the broader politics of genomic biobanking. Some of the ethical literature concerning the establishment of biobanking in Africa echoes the well-established trope of genetic diversity (see also Chaps. 3 and 5) as a benefit for biobanking, but also points to the exploitative North-South relations that have shaped much medical research on the continent (Dandara et al., 2014; Staunton & de Vries, 2020). African biobanking initiatives such as the Human Heredity and Health in Africa (H3Africa) consortium therefore put much weight on avoiding exploitation through the engagement of local communities and building domestic research capacity (Amoakoh-Coleman et al., 2023; Dandara et al., 2014). Nevertheless, some observers point to the limitations of and differences between existing (national) governance frameworks and ethical guidelines for biobanking in Africa (Tindana et al., 2019). More specifically, and in spite of expressed concerns over exploitation, certain ethicists argue for less restrictive regulations in order to allow sharing and so-called secondary use of materials stored in African biobanks (Staunton & de Vries, 2020; de Vries et al., 2017). What this brief excursion demonstrates, then, is how established ethical arguments (e.g., for 'broad' consent that allows materials donated for one study to be used in others) overlap with, but may not necessarily address issues of (global) inequality and marginalization. Myness Kasanda Ndambo and colleagues (Ndambo et al., 2024) therefore emphasize how seemingly non-invasive (physical) sampling can be socially invasive, as it interferes with cultural understandings of body materials, fears of exploitation and forms of trust based on misconceptions of the direct therapeutic value of research participation. More profound engagement with the purposes of medical tissue and data collection project and how they materialize in both the organization and conduct of research is therefore required.

In their book on biobank governance, Herbert Gottweis and Alan Petersen (2008) have described this complex domain in terms of the interrelated governance *of* and governance *through* biobanks. They use this distinction to describe how, on the one hand, biobanks and biobanking practices are shaped by organizational, regulatory, ethical and other preconditions while, on the other, particular configurations of biobanks shape our understandings of life, health and disease and the affiliated rights and responsibilities attributed to human individuals and collectives. Biobanks are thereby subjects of both the politics of science and what Nikolas Rose (2001) might term "the politics of life itself". Biobanks thereby form a particularly interesting lens for looking at the ways scientific knowledge on human life, ways of knowing life, and rights and responsibilities with regard to health and disease jointly get constituted (Jasanoff, 2011). More specifically, such collections also embody manifestations of how such relations between life and rights are imagined to be constructed in medical research (Hurlbut et al., 2020). Rather than studying these implications in terms of abstract ethical principles, though, understanding governance of and through biobanks requires more grounded empirical analysis of how different biobanking (or broadly tissue and data collection) projects work. Such analysis should extend from organization and financing through collection, processing, storage and use of materials on to the social circulation and implications of research results—covering the full 'lifespan' of biobanking (Aarden, 2024).

The interconnections between governance of and through medical research are obviously not exclusive to biobanking. Barbara Prainsack (2017, 2018), for example, has warned against understanding the individual as an atomistic entity in the context of personalized medicine, arguing that even health care tailored to the single person requires practices of solidarity to reduce inequalities. Equally focusing on the prominence of individual risks and ideas of magic bullet cures in global health, for example, João Biehl and Adriana Petryna (2013) have described how the funding and institutionalization of research shape an approach to evidence that fails to account for the complexity of disease. Adele Clarke et al. (2010) have proposed an overarching analytic for this increased reliance on technoscience in medicine in terms of biomedicalization. They diagnose both a material transformation of medicine and an extension of its jurisdiction to ever more domains of life as key processes of change. These various examples each present diagnoses of an increasing focus on technoscientific meanings of health and disease associated with particular regulatory and organizational configurations in terms of, for instance, biocapital (Sunder Rajan, 2006), philantrocapitalism (McGoey, 2015; Global Health Watch, 2011) and a move away from the nation state in relation to the promises of data-centric medical research (Cool, 2016).[3]

Particularly feminist and postcolonial approaches in science and technology studies (STS) have long identified the asymmetries and inequalities that result from scientific knowledge "[emerging] as a central actor and tool for state and global projects" (Pollock & Subramaniam, 2016, p. 952). Sandra Harding (2006), for example, has cast doubt on the idea that science equals social progress by pointing to the particular, often far from egalitarian, values embedded in science and technology. Harding argues that science has historically often reproduced and reinforced existing inequalities. She has pointed out how "...technical, cognitive elements of scientific practices and the information they produce always represent social and political priorities, meanings and ideas as well as more or less accurate pictures of nature's order" (Harding, 2006, p. 116). This position implies once more that consideration of the normative dimensions of science ought to consider more than merely the ethics of scientific conduct.

Ruha Benjamin (2013), for example, has considered these issues in her study of public funding for stem cell research in California. She demonstrates how "features of the present that systematically prevent health and wealth gains from 'trickling down' to the masses" are often not considered in such future-oriented research initiatives (Benjamin, 2013, p. 13). It is not self-evident that the disadvantaged benefit from scientific progress, which raises the question if and how commitments to speculative science relate to notions of the public good. This question is all the more pressing, so she argues, in light of socioeconomic inequalities that make those who are likely to benefit the least from technological advancements most likely to do the "clinical labour" (Cooper & Waldby, 2014) of donation and participation in and for research. Under those circumstances, ethical principles that protect research participants in the abstract are not sufficient to fully avoid exploitation.

In recognition of the shortcomings of a narrow and principled understanding of ethics, then, social scientists have turned to justice as an alternative. The notion of justice can be used to confront the values embedded in scientific and technological projects directly and to account for how these embedded values affect both individuals and collectives. Yet scholars in STS have also noted the heterogeneity of the concept of justice as well as how justice can itself be part of scientific legitimation strategies—and thus become an object of analysis as well as an objective to pursue (Mamo & Fishman, 2013). Jenny Reardon (2013, 2017), for example, has pointed out how the pursuit of justice has become part of the repertoire for legitimating genomics, for example in the form of claims that a focus on genomic factors in disease may help to redress historical injustices. While such claims promote values of inclusiveness and universalism through the sharing of data, they obscure ongoing exclusions and asymmetries in biomedical research.

Postcolonial and feminist studies of science and technology have addressed such asymmetries in both the institutionalization of science and the construction and valuation of knowledge focusing, for example, on the intersections between science and the (post)colonial state and hierarchies of different forms of knowledge (Subramaniam et al., 2017). While feminism and postcolonialism may focus on different (yet intersecting) realms of inequality, Sandra Harding (2009, p. 418) has highlighted how both "decenter and parochialize dominant ways of thinking about the production of scientific and technological knowledge and their familiar philosophical assumptions". In doing so, Harding (2009, p. 403) maintains, "feminism and postcolonialism both argue in effect that how we live together both enables and limits what we can know, and vice versa". Knowledge is thus always shaped by the circumstances of its production, while simultaneously shaping its circumstances of application. Scientific knowledge thereby both reflects and reproduces existing inequalities and thus has profound social significance. This is also the case for medical research and genomics where, in spite of claims towards the end of race and a shift towards a focus on populations, existing racial categories continue to be used and racial inequalities in health and access to medicine continue to exist (Kowal, 2022; Pollock, 2012). For medical research collections, feminist and postcolonial studies of science thus strongly suggest that the intricacies of scientific practice and governance have to be considered to lay bare how they shape and are shaped by particular normative commitments.

In addition to the persistent inequalities engrained in the production and public application of scientific knowledge, postcolonial studies of science have highlighted how imagined differences across geographies as well as persistent material and political marginalizations get reproduced *within science itself* (Anderson, 2009; Prasad, 2014a). Such work suggests that social studies of science need to be attentive to global power imbalances. Shiv Visvanathan (2002, p. 92) has therefore described STS as "a creative meditation on the relation between knowledge and power". He further writes that to make sense of this relation, the field needs to be "conceptually ambidextrous. It needs both a theory of knowledge and of politics" (Visvanathan, 2002, p. 97). Although his argument primarily pertains to the plurality of forms of knowledge and a striving for "cognitive justice" (Visvanathan, 2005), my aim is to develop the heuristic of *infrastructures for the purpose of population-based medical research* to make sense of the production of both knowledge and power in medical research collections. More particularly, I build on the preceding discussion of promises, practices, governance and justice in medical research collections to centre the question how such infrastructure jointly produce knowledge and exercise power in the sense of defining which meanings of health and disease matter and are prioritized—in research and beyond. I will now turn to my own approach in studying these infrastructures, before sketching out some primary contours of the analytical heuristic I develop further in subsequent chapters.

Towards an Analytical Heuristic: Four Cases

My analysis of four infrastructures for the purpose of population-based medical research builds on some of the key insights from the literature on biomedical research collections and biobanks in particular that I have discussed previously. These infrastructures all embody particular promises of specific forms of value—which may be scientific, economic or otherwise—that are pursued through the particular configuration of research practices and the organization, regulation and funding of these infrastructures (which I try to capture with the term governance). A key aspect of these infrastructures, then, is that their particular purposes consist of benefits envisioned for particular populations, to be produced through both or either of the organizational configuration of tissue and data collection as such and/or the forms of knowledge produced therein. Drawing on postcolonial and feminist studies of science and technology, I further seek to excavate the normative commitments embedded within the way knowledge production is organized and practised. More precisely, I focus on how these commitments were built into the making of and subsequent reshaping of infrastructures as referred to by the notion of infrastructuring (Star & Ruhleder, 1996; Karasti & Blomberg, 2018). This notion emphasizes how infrastructure is never completed and never static. Focusing on infrastructuring across four different case studies means that I further develop the different elements of my analytical heuristic—infrastructure, purpose, population and medical research—through an in-depth discussion of one case study each, while simultaneously keeping an eye on the normative dimensions built into these infrastructures.

The case studies in Chaps. 2, 3, 4, and 5 were conducted over a timespan of nearly a decade on the basis of a combination of qualitative research methods, using a range of materials (see Table 1.1). Since I focused on the approaches to knowledge production and purposes envisioned in the set-up of each of these collection efforts, I studied public performances of these cases rather than knowledge production processes as such. My study is therefore not an ethnography of scientific work or even of research governance. It does incorporate ethnographic

Table 1.1 Overview of the materials collected by case study

Case	Materials
Framingham Heart Study	• Interviews with eight study collaborators and government officials • Primary study literature, including scientific publications, intermediary reports, etc. • Secondary literature on history and organization of the study
Singapore Tissue Network	• Interviews with 13 staff members of STN and research institutions and government officials • Publications on biomedical sciences in Singapore in *Science* and *Nature* affiliated journals • Publications on biobanks in Singapore newspapers • Observations at a biobank staff meeting and two 'science & society' public events
Million Death Study	• Interviews with 13 researchers and government officials • Study protocols, manuals and guidelines • Publications on study aims, methods and results (via PubMed)
BBMRI-ERIC	• Interviews with 13 BBMRI-ERIC staff members and other key actors • BBMRI-ERIC publications including annual reports, work programmes, newsletters and formal documents • Observation at three *Europe Biobank Week* conferences and webinars

sensitivities in exploring how study researchers and administrators (understood broadly to also include, for example, policy-makers not directly involved in these collection initiatives as such) narrated and gave meaning to, for example, study recruitment, methods, aims, sample and data collection efforts, etc. My approach resonates with the idea of combining the study of technoscientific and institutional practices Ayo Wahlberg (2022) describes as "assemblage ethnography". He emphasizes how contemporary technological societies are shaped by interrelated practices of knowledge production and governance that take place across different scales, sites and practices. Assemblage ethnography, then, has informed my understanding of how the kinds of sociotechnical configurations I am interested in come to operate in the world.

Against this background, the collection of data I used consisted primarily of interviews and the analysis of both formal (study) documents and representations of the various collection initiatives in both scientific and general media (e.g., scientific journals, newspapers). This data collection took on slightly different form in each case study, due to both differences between the case studies as such and between the various ways I was able to engage. Interview respondents were mostly identified directly through publicly accessible information about the case studies such as institutional websites or scientific publications as well as through further contacts suggested by initial respondents. I studied documents both as public representations of the various studies as well as—where relevant—as actors shaping the collection initiatives themselves (e.g., in the form of study manuals) (Shankar et al., 2017). On a few occasions, I had the opportunity to do more classic ethnographic work in the form of observations at public events, although this mostly informed my ability to situate a case study in its wider scientific, social and political environment.

In my analysis of the collected materials, I was largely guided by the mapping approach developed by Adele Clarke and colleagues (2005, 2015) in terms of situational analysis. I took as key insights from this approach to, one, consider the situation under analysis as a construction made by the researcher and, two, map the positions of and relations between different actors as the main move in reconstructing social reality. This meant that I cut off my analysis at particular points that shape how I describe them. I made three analytical decisions in this regard, which may also amount to shortcomings in my analysis. The first of these was, as indicated before, to focus less on actual research practices and more on narratives of operation, purpose and outcome. My second decision has been to focus on the case studies at particular points in time, which means that some more recent developments (for example changes to the European biobanking infrastructure BBMRI-ERIC under their current, third Director-General; see Chap. 5) have not been taken into account. Finally, I decided to not extend my analysis too far beyond what I consider the core of these initiatives. In doing so, I reduced complexity in the interest of being able to draw some comparative conclusions that I think are informative for thinking through 'big' medical research at present.

The selection of the four case studies I introduce in more detail shortly was based on a number of relatively loose criteria. Not least among them was my desire to explore how 'global' dimensions of biomedical research touched ground in particular places in the early twenty-first century. Admittedly, some of this initial interest got lost along the way—I would have written a different book if that had not been the case. But it informed my interest in cases that both cover a range of geographical locations as well as medical research beyond the domain of genomic biobanking alone. This, then, has been a second consideration—to see if and how 'pre-'(as opposed to post-)genomic collection initiatives would be similar or different. Third, the initiatives discussed here have in common that they have (largely) been funded by public means and are managed and coordinated by public agencies—although neither of these characteristics is absolute in any of these cases. Certain aspects of funding and implementations of each of these collections are or have been covered—or are/were expected to be covered—by financial resources from, for example, private companies or philanthropic organizations. Similarly, what 'public' means in terms of funding, coordination, implementation, etc. may differ substantially and include anything from national health and science ministries directly, to competitive research grants, to routine public services contributing to these collections. Finally, as I proceeded with this research, I increasingly found the assumption that any of them served to produce a nebulous public good of particular interest.

In each of the four chapters that address a particular case study, I aim to refine my analytical heuristic on the basis of empirical insight into the practices, governance and value commitments of tissue and data collection and knowledge production.

In the next chapter, I explore the meaning of *infrastructures* for medical research through an analysis of the Framingham Heart Study. This study is named after the town in the northeastern United States where it started in the late 1940s to study the "stresses and insults of various types" contributing to heart disease (Gordon & Kannel, 1968, p. 1b-3). The study has persisted ever since, and has entered medical lore as "probably the most celebrated epidemiological study in the history of medicine and public health" (Roberts, 2000, p. 106). While its original focus was on tracing if and to what extent certain behaviours increased the likelihood that people would contract certain forms of cardiovascular disease, later efforts involved the study of familial and genetic factors based on the inclusion of a second and third generation of participants (Kannel et al.,

1979; Splansky et al., 2007). The study thus has the reputation to have contributed significantly to critical methodological developments in contemporary epidemiology; however, historians and social science analysts of medicine have expressed critiques of the narrow behavioural focus of the 'risk factor' concept emerging from the study (Rothstein, 2003) and the equally narrowly conceived cohorts of mainly white European descent. The Framingham Heart Study, which was originally conceived as a 20-year project that persisted as a result of strategic methodological innovations once it neared the end of its original funding period (Patel, 2012), is thus an important marker for medical population research in the twentieth century.

Since the study was conceived from the very beginning as "a continuing resource for the study of cardiovascular disease" (Gordon & Kannel, 1968, p. 1a-1), it provides a useful case for exploring medical research collections as infrastructure. An important strand of social science analysis of infrastructures stresses how they are often taken for granted in their everyday operations, becoming visible only when they malfunction (Star, 1999). Here, infrastructures are conceived as "prior work [...] that supports and enables the activity we are really engaged in doing" (Slota & Bowker, 2017, p. 529). This is certainly one aspect of tissue and data collections for research, where the collection work is often done in preparation for work on specific scientific questions that are not always specified initially. The Framingham Heart Study is a case in point; while it began with quite specific questions, once data on its cohort had been collected for a longer span of time and subsequent cohorts were added, it provided a basis for still other questions to be investigated. At the same time, various analysts have pointed out how infrastructures are not exclusively functional and often anything but invisible (Larkin, 2013; Anand et al., 2018). Infrastructures are often imbued with promises and imaginaries of progress. This, too, is a dimension of the Framingham Study, which is reflected in both how researchers discuss its success in terms of the relations build up with participants over time, and in the aforementioned status the study has obtained as an exemplar of modern epidemiological research. Regardless of whether the functional invisibility or performative visibility of infrastructures are emphasized, however, analysts agree that infrastructures are quintessentially political "sociotechnical ensembles" (Bijker, 1995). Translated to the context of medical research collections, this political dimension follows from the ways particular configurations of what is collected and stored, from whom, and how, has effects on how specific definitions of health, risk and responsibility get articulated. In the case of the Framingham Heart Study, this aspect entails not only the focus on behavioural risks and racial bias, but also the longitudinal persistence of such effects as the study's particular approach to heart disease continues.

Chapter 3 is concerned with the idea of the *purpose* of medical research, which I address through the case of the Singapore Tissue Network. This network was formed through the centralized storage of tissues collected in the context of government-funded medical research projects in Singapore. It was established as one of several support infrastructures that were part of a large-scale investment in setting up a biomedical research sector in the country around the turn of the Millennium (Cyranoski, 2001; Clancey, 2012). This sector was explicitly imagined in economic terms as an opportunity to both develop domestic capabilities in biotechnology and pharmaceutical innovation and to attract foreign life science companies to Singapore. As such, this Biomedical Sciences Initiative (BMSI), and the Singapore Tissue Network along with it were to foreground Singapore as both representative of different populations in Asia and as a bridgehead to access the potentially vast Asian biomedical market (Ong, 2015; Fischer, 2013). However, the Singapore Tissue Network was short-lived (Chan, 2012). While one influential explanation for its fate was to point to the lack of use of stored materials by medical researchers, this reasoning obscures underlying issues with how the network was conceived. What turned out to be a fundamental flaw for the Singapore Tissue Network was a disagreement between policy objectives and scientists' beliefs on how such a repository could become useful (Aarden, 2017b). While this was largely an implicit disagreement, it shaped how the network was designed on the one hand and (not) used on the other.

The fate of the Singapore Tissue Network thus points to how a tissue and data repository may have various purposes to different groups of involved actors. I approach these different perceptions of the network's value from two theoretical angles. On the one hand, a tissue repository as a support structure for economically productive medical research reflects a (sociotechnical) imaginary (Jasanoff & Kim, 2015; McNeil et al., 2017) of how science can contribute to social progress. This imaginary informed investments in biomedical research in Singapore and was as such largely accepted by biobanking practitioners. Underlying understandings of and approaches to the making of value from stored materials, however, ultimately diverged. Following analyses of how value gets made in practices (Dussauge et al., 2015a), the case of the Singapore Tissue Network shows how limited use of stored materials was itself an outcome of different perceptions of how materials can be made valuable. These differences largely revolved around questions of collaboration. Whereas the design of the Singapore Tissue Network was based on the assumption that collaboration would result from making high quality materials available, many researchers felt that more established relationships of familiarity and trust were required for them to want to work with (materials contributed by) others.

My focus in Chap. 4 is on the notion of *population*, and specifically how populations get captured in data, on the basis of the Million Death Study in India. This study was set up as an alternative to the arguably defective civil mortality registration system in India and was intended to generate more accurate statistics on the distribution of causes of death in the country. In typical global health fashion, it maps health, disease and death within national borders in the global South based on resources contributed by a range of institutions (Crane, 2010; McGoey et al., 2011). The particular innovation advanced in the Million Death Study is to rely on an existing, representative demographic population sample and door-to-door collection of symptomatic data—a method described as verbal autopsy (VA)—to be able to, first, determine individual causes of death and, second, aggregate these into causal national mortality statistics (Jha et al., 2006; Vogel, 2012). An aspect of particular interest about this study is how different versions of the Indian population—as a research sample, as an aggregate of causes of death, but also as a regionally and socioeconomically differentiated collective—get produced through and with different 'datafication' technologies (Mejias & Couldry, 2019). In the Million Death Study, these technologies do not necessarily take the shape of digital data technologies, and yet they incorporate logics of the present "data revolution" (Kitchin, 2014b) in interesting ways. Closer analysis of the study thereby provides insight into how a population becomes data become diagnoses become a population again.

How populations are defined and turned into numbers has been a long-standing interest in social science research (Curtis, 2002; Foucault, 2007; Saetnan et al., 2011; Cool, 2022), particularly in the context of colonial intersections between knowledge and power. The census is the exemplary technology in this regard (Cohn, 1987), and one of the key characteristics of the Million Death Study is how it relies on a quantification infrastructure that is associated with the census. It thereby seeks to correct shortcomings of the state in one domain by relying on a different state infrastructure. More precisely, a core motivation for setting up this study has been a critique of the malfunctioning of the Indian state in matters pertaining to public health; at the same time, study researchers consider the state's demographic infrastructure inescapable for collecting data with the scale and consistency required for a reliable mortality survey. This implies that 'knowing' the population and its causes of death through a range of data technologies (ranging from software platforms to diagnostic and data collection guidelines) is also related to particular variations of the state and its effectiveness in governing (aspects of) a population's collective lives. Put differently, attending to population health in India in the context of the Million Death Study includes and entangles both micro practices of data generation, collection and processing, and broader processes of imagining governance and the state's responsibilities. As part of this process, individual diagnoses need to be produced and classified (Bowker & Star, 1999) in ways that balance a desire for diagnostic accuracy with the limitations of deficient civil registration and the aim of improving health policy.

Chapter 5 is about the various meanings *medical research* may have, which I investigate in relation to the European Biobanking and Biomolecular Resources Research Infrastructure—European Research Infrastructure Consortium (BBMRI-ERIC). This "research infrastructure", which holds this designation on account of its formal legal recognition as such under European Union law, is by and large a product of European science policy in the early twenty-first century (Lauss, 2009; Vuorio, 2017). While the idea of building a network of existing tissue and data repositories in different EU member states made scientific sense in light of the larger cohorts of research subjects required for research "after the genome" (Yuille et al., 2007), the initial steps towards building such a network were taken in the context of an EU-funded research project. As the EU further pursued a strategy of building large-scale, collaborative and often distributed research infrastructures, BBMRI (which only later added the clause—ERIC to designate its formal legal recognition) got stabilized and formalized in line with this strategy. As a result BBMRI-ERIC is presently a scientific-political hybrid that defines its membership in terms of both individual biobanks and nation states (Aarden, 2025). It has built out a number of services to biobanks and research institutions, which include platforms for finding and accessing samples and data and support on ethical and legal questions, while simultaneously navigating fluctuations in membership and national governments' willingness to pay. Whereas the infrastructure's growing membership is considered to be a sign of success at least in terms of size, some of the people involved express concern about its contributions to enhancing medical research in Europe. This latter concern points to the question how, exactly, research infrastructures relate to medical research practice.

Two key aspects of the questions what medical research *is* and what it is *for* are at the centre of the discourse around BBMRI-ERIC. The question of the infrastructure's role in medical research, then, is articulated along various axes related to both questions of European integration and of the organization of medical research. The dimension of European integration takes on the shape of, for example, questions regarding the building of European infrastructures vis-à-vis funding for more specific research projects as well as with regard to the relations between the European infrastructure, nation states and individual biobanks. Standards are a central element in efforts to integrate biobanking in Europe, but do not necessarily harmonize practices of, for example, quality management and sample accessibility (cf. Timmermans & Epstein, 2010). Furthermore, the question of science's economic significance and contribution to European integration (Benner, 2018) features prominently in debates about both strategic reorientations of the infrastructure and its success (or lack thereof) in doing what it was supposed to do. Medical research thereby can take on a number of different shapes and meanings depending on how its relation to established challenges of European integration is perceived (Von Hirschhausen & Patel, 2010).

In Chap. 6, I draw the four cases together to further develop my analytical heuristic. Whereas I discuss different aspect on the basis of individual cases in the preceding chapters, I argue here that the notion of infrastructures for the purpose of population-based medical research as a whole can help make sense of the value commitments that inform each of the four collection initiatives. Jointly, they further provide insight into key dimensions of and developments in contemporary research in health and disease, such as questions of a developing bioeconomy, the emergence of 'big data' and changing interactions between science and society. These insights suggest that there are certain shared characteristics between these cases, which raises the question how and why to compare them (Jasanoff, 2005). That question in turn invites a methodological reflection in which I argue for thick comparison and juxtaposition as strategies for illuminating normative differences between cases without essentializing them.

I finally return to the question of public goods and participation in the concluding chapter. To address the question who benefits from medical research, I propose to engage with discussions of biological and social citizenship in relation to medical research (Rose & Novas, 2005; Laruffa, 2022). I will argue that a particular conception of citizenship can be distilled from each of the case studies, which provides insight into how rights and responsibilities of both individual and collective research participants as well as broader populations are conceived. From this observation I once more turn to the question of participation in its dual meaning of contributing to research and to its governance (Tutton, 2007). I draw on STS discussions of public engagement with science to highlight some of its limitations in the context of medical research (Irwin, 2015; Chilvers & Kearnes, 2016). Instead, I argue that the deep normative commitments embedded in medical research collections require a broader democratic approach—including considerations of value commitments in science—to participation and the governance of research.

Notes

1. For a discussion of the biobank metaphor, see (Cho et al., 2018).
2. But, for a critique of too loose a definition of biobanks, see (Annaratone et al., 2021).
3. For somewhat older and possibly more fundamental critiques of increasingly technical understandings of health and disease, see also (Illich, 1975; Kothari & Mehta, 1988).

2

Building Heart Disease Research as Infrastructure in the Framingham Heart Study

In the Winter of 2012/2013, I visited the Framingham Heart Study (FHS) intramural clinic in the town of Framingham, a few dozen kilometres west of Boston in the northeastern United States (US). Located in a rather non-descript concrete office building, the clinic was quiet on this particular day. As a researcher showed me the labs and examination rooms, a study nurse lamented that all appointments on this snowy day had been cancelled. As my host explained, this was in part due to the point in the examination cycle at which the study had landed. About two-thirds through the examination of all study participants, which included three generations of cohorts at the time, the people scheduled to come to the clinic would be those who either had busy schedules or no longer lived in or near Framingham itself—and who would thus be more likely to cancel. Yet, my host was quick to point out that there is more to the Framingham Study than the regular examination of study participants. Examination results and (mainly blood) samples collected over more than six (by now seven) decades were available for continued analysis. As another researcher would surmise in a later interview, 'Framingham' (the name of the town having become equivalent for the multi-decade research effort) can be understood as a repository for novel research related to cardiovascular disease, much of it done by research groups

E. Aarden, *Producing Citizenship in Medical Research Collections*, Health, Technology and Society, https://doi.org/10.1007/978-981-95-1707-7_2

elsewhere. The data and materials, so Framingham Study researchers argued, are available to be shared—and supposedly drawing significant interest from around the world.

The widespread interest in Framingham samples and data is undoubtedly related to its outsized reputation as one of the earliest and most influential epidemiological studies of cardiovascular disease (see, e.g., Roberts, 2000). In a rather celebratory history co-written by one of the former study directors, for example, the study is characterized as a quiet revolution, through which "its researchers refashioned cardiovascular disease epidemiology in ways that revolutionized medicine" (Levy & Brink, 2005, p. 8). Others, too, have characterized the Framingham Study as highly influential in the history of medical research in the twentieth century, pointing to two decisive contributions to the contemporary understanding of cardiovascular conditions. On the one hand, the development of an epidemiological notion of "risk factors" for disease, attributed to the Framingham Study, has been characterized as the "outstanding single achievement" of cardiovascular epidemiology (Epstein, 1992, p. 25). On the other hand, the study's methodological approach of a prospective study of a randomized population sample is considered a key innovation for the discipline of epidemiology.

Beyond the domains of cardiovascular disease and epidemiological research, the Framingham Study can arguably be considered a salient example of broader trends towards "biomedicalization" (Clarke et al., 2010) in the second half of the twentieth century. It thereby reflects broader transformations in the social meaning of health and disease that increasingly highlight (largely) asymptomatic disease risks and the detrimental effects of individual lifestyle. Other examples of this shift include, for example, the changing relation between smoking and health (Brandt, 2007) and the emergence of preventive pharmacology to treat early signs of future disease (Greene, 2007). The Framingham Heart Study is thereby a significant example of changes in medicine in the twentieth century and the building of associated research infrastructures.

At the same time, the Framingham Study and what it implies for contemporary understandings of health and disease has been widely critiqued. Both the lack of attention for diversity in its original 'random' sample and the implications of a perspective on risk framed in terms of individual behaviour have been scrutinized by social scientists and historians. In her study of how difference comes to matter in the meanings attributed to heart disease, for example, Janet Shim (2014) highlights how the retrospective narrative of the innovative character of the Framingham Study has obscured concerns about generalizability and representativeness of the study's results. These concerns have lingering effects on epidemiological studies, including on those aimed at addressing the lack of diversity in the Framingham cohorts. Historian Robert Aronowitz has pointed to the narrow, individualized view of disease promoted through "discrete, mechanism-driven risk factors" (Aronowitz, 1998, pp. 108–109) that gives part of its social meaning to cardiovascular disease. Furthermore, the notion of risk factor, which originated from the life insurance industry, has taken on a different meaning in the context of the Framingham Study. To make the notion useful to clinical practice, risk factors are often considered in isolation, and a host of potential risks—particularly related to social issues such as education level, income, marital status and the like—have not been considered in the original study set-up (Rothstein, 2003). The medical notion of risk factor developed in the Framingham Study thereby promotes a very particular view of disease that has since been carried forward over more than half a century of further research.

In this chapter, I focus on how the Framingham Heart Study's particular framing of epidemiological research has afforded and restricted particular forms of research on cardiovascular disease. This includes the study's present status as a repository from which samples and data get circulated for the purpose of (primarily) genomic research. I argue that this line of inquiry can be made productive by thinking of the Framingham Study as an *infrastructure* for medical research. This perspective draws in part on studies of how scientific laboratories "reconfigure" research objects in order to generate scientific truth claims (Knorr-Cetina, 1999; Latour & Woolgar, 1986), which point to the sociomaterial complexity of scientific practice. Yet, the notion of infrastructure moves further to take seriously the view expressed in a report on the initial 20-year duration of the Framingham Study that described the study as "a continuing resource for the study of cardiovascular disease" (Gordon & Kannel, 1968, p. 1). Written at a moment when, as we will see, continuation of the study was not self-evident, this particular statement points out how thinking through the study as an infrastructure ties its past and future together (Appel et al., 2018). The processes through which the

Framingham Heart Study became and was maintained as infrastructure can be described as an ongoing process of *infrastructuring*. A focus on infrastructuring allows making the connections that enabled and maintained a particular approach to cardiovascular disease research visible. Thus, to paraphrase Susan Leigh Star's (Star & Ruhleder, 1996; Star, 1999) influential work on infrastructures, it shows relations to be at the heart of what infrastructure is. Often invisible, infrastructures make other forms of work possible by arranging existing things in new ways (Slota & Bowker, 2017). Infrastructures often remain in the background and persist, changing only incrementally. However, this is not always the case, as infrastructures can also be made (deliberately) visible, iconic even, and be tied to political promises and collective desires (Larkin, 2013, 2018).

Below, I trace how the notion of infrastructure makes visible what the particular organizational and epistemic configuration of the Framingham Heart Study has made possible and imaginable in cardiovascular epidemiology, as well as where it renders particular research questions and approaches more challenging to pursue. In the next section I provide a brief historical overview of the study from its origins to the present, in order to illustrate the infrastructuring of cardiovascular epidemiology. Next, I turn to how the study infrastructure has been made visible and has been projected as a landmark for medical research, while particular characteristics of the study have also become iconic in shaping imaginations of ways forward within the study itself. Finally, I trace how organizational and epistemic affordances of the study infrastructure together with imaginations of what makes this infrastructure work shape current research practices in the Framingham Study, with a particular focus on the exploration of genetic factors in cardiovascular disease.

Establishing and Maintaining a Cardiovascular Disease Research Infrastructure

Over the decades, it has become a central part of the Framingham Study's iconography to point to an emerging "epidemic" of cardiovascular disease after the Second World War as a key inspiration for the study, and to Framingham as an "average" American town to explain why the study was started there (Levy & Brink, 2005; Gehlbach, 2005). Although there may be some legitimacy to these claims, several other characteristics of medical research policy and practice around the middle of the twentieth century have been equally important. For one, the years immediately following the Second World War saw an increased interest in the public funding of science in general, and of medical research in particular in the United States. As a growing health problem that seemed to be associated with growing wealth and consumption, cardiovascular disease drew considerable interest in the post-war years. Efforts to use the growing interest in medical research to study this complex of health conditions then ended up being located in Framingham at least in part as a matter of convenience. The vicinity of Framingham to the institutional home of various promoters of the study of heart disease in the Boston area undoubtedly plaid as much a role as the averageness of the town (Levy & Brink, 2005). That said, certain characteristics of Framingham as "a meat-and-potatoes kind of place" (Gehlbach, 2005, p. 210) did play a role.[1] When the study started, the size of the town, together with previous involvement in a study of tuberculosis and the presence of various local forms of voluntary organization were thought to be indicative of the likelihood of the local population's continued participation in the study.

The making of an infrastructure can be characterized as an "ontological experiment" to emphasize how new states of the world and relations between actors are made through processes of infrastructuring (Bruun Jensen & Morita, 2015). New infrastructures in science can change definitions of what knowledge is and how it is generated (Jackson & Barbrow, 2013) and thereby be sites of conflict, identity formation and distribution all at once before the infrastructure becomes self-evident (Jackson et al., 2007). In the early years of the Framingham Study, we may see such volatility in the involvement of various institutions that each brought their own understanding of how heart disease ought to be studied. In spite of retrospective emphasis on the study's methodological innovations (Gehlbach, 2005), the initial purposes of the Framingham Study included early detection and screening for heart disease as well as efforts to control the spread of disease. The initial study population consisted of volunteers and the study was coordinated by the United States Public Health Service (Levy & Brink, 2005; Dawber, 1980; Oppenheimer, 2005, 2010). After a few years, coordination and management of the study were transferred to the newly established National Heart Institute (NHI; presently the National Heart, Lung, and Blood Institute—NHLBI), part of the National Institutes of Health. As commonly told, the shift to this institute implied a strengthened emphasis on scientific rigour—which refers to the recruitment of a randomly selected population cohort and the prospective study of disease. The study had started with recruiting volunteers, which illustrates how infrastructure started out as a form of experiment (Bruun Jensen & Morita, 2015)—with lasting effects, since the voluntary participants remained part of the study cohort. The study would focus on "the investigation of change over time and its determinants" (Dwyer & Feinleib, 1992, p. 5) via regular examination of participants to see if they developed cardiovascular disease and to (potentially) link that observation to particular characteristics and behaviours.

The study approach that to some extent came together coincidentally stabilized over the originally planned 20 years the study would run. So did its particular understanding of 'determinants' of heart disease. Starting from the idea that "stresses and insults of various types" would, over time, result in a number of study participants developing cardiovascular disease (Gordon & Kannel, 1968, p. 3), the study started with defining a number of hypotheses linking particular (possible) causes to specific effects. This required defining criteria for measuring both contributing factors or causes, disease outcomes and the link between them.[2] As an example of criteria for disease outcomes, the coronary condition angina pectoris was defined as:

> Brief recurrent chest discomfort of up to 15 minutes duration, precipitated by exertion or emotion and relieved by rest or by nitro-glycerine, was regarded as angina pectoris (AP) if two physicians interviewing the subject agreed that this condition was definitely present. This diagnosis was based on evaluation of a subjective manifestation; no post-exercise ECG abnormality or ECG abnormality at rest was required. (Feinleib et al., 1968, p. 2)

Similarly, alcohol consumption as a possible 'stress or insult' contributing to CVD was measured such:

> The use of alcoholic beverages by the subject was recorded by the examining physician on the medical history form at Exam 2, 4, and 7. The information consisted of three items:
>
> A = average number of highballs or cocktails per 30-day month
> B = average number of 8-ounce glasses of beer per 30-day month
> C = average number of 4-ounce glasses of wine per 30-day month
>
> To compute the equivalent alcohol in ounces per month this formula was used:
>
> $$\text{Alcohol} = 1.00\ \text{A} + 0.40\ \text{B} + 0.67\ \text{C}$$
>
> This was done only for subjects with details on all three items (A, B, and C) in the history form. (Cole et al., 1974)

For alcohol consumption, the questionnaire at the aforementioned examinations included questions whether individuals were currently consuming alcohol or had done so in the past, and if so, how many cocktails or glasses of beer or wine they drank per day and how many days per month. Over the course of the study, answers to these questions were parsed by sex and age groups to be able to say, for example, which percentage of men aged 50–60 with an alcohol consumption of 7 (according to the formula above) developed angina—and thus to determine whether alcohol consumption significantly raises the likelihood of this condition.

These criteria show how specific inscriptions (Latour & Woolgar, 1986) of disease and contributing factors feature into the building of an infrastructure. Defining what angina pectoris and alcohol consumption—or, for that matter, stroke and high blood pressure—mean and how it can be measured form a prerequisite for all the other work to be done in the study. This work includes the identification of people who meet specific criteria, matching different criteria and aggregating many of such matches to gain insight into correlations, and possible causal relations. Inscriptions are thereby infrastructural to the study and, once defined, thereby shape which kinds of questions a study can answer or not. In a study that continued for as long as the Framingham Heart Study, such inscriptions are recalibrated when new techniques get introduced, yet continue to leave traces and circumscribe the range of available research options.

The formulation of hypotheses around particular factors contributing to the endpoints of disease shows how knowledge production in the study is infrastructured in particular ways. First, the hypotheses included in the study largely focused on individual behaviours and lifestyle—smoking, alcohol consumption, physical activity, diet and the like. The FHS was therefore from the beginning predisposed to finding causes in the behavioural realm. This is—in part—a result of focusing the investigation on questions and hypotheses considered acceptable to the local community (Gordon & Kannel, 1968). Second, although the very approach of the study meant that it would take a number of years before any reliable results could be expected, the idea that lifestyle factors were key was quite established from early on (Oppenheimer, 2010). Finally, the study had a relatively high retention rate. According to an NHI report, between 75% and 80% of the cohort participated in all of the first eight examinations—with the continued participation, perhaps unsurprisingly, highest among volunteers and most of the drop-out occurring between exams one and two. Furthermore, 531 people had died in the meantime. These deaths were remarkably described as losses to follow-up, yet valued positively for staying in the study until reaching the ultimate end point (Gordon, 1968, p. 2). These notes on definitions of diagnostic criteria, data comparison and participant retention show how the early phase of the study was largely about building an infrastructure. This infrastructure, in turn, not only rested on institutions, but also involved study participants and particular ways of knowing.

After several rounds of examination, first results of the study began to be published by the late 1950s. Yet, retrospectively, a 1961 paper with the title *Factors of Risk in the Development of Coronary Heart Disease* (Kannel et al., 1961) has been highlighted as the landmark publication launching the understanding of heart disease in terms of risk factors (Levy & Brink, 2005). This paper describes how a combination of characteristics—high blood pressure, raised cholesterol and a electrocardiographic pattern of left ventricular hypertrophy—both individually, but especially in combination, significantly raise a person's risk of developing coronary heart disease. The paper therefore argues that identification of these three characteristics "allows the identification of the coronary prone individual many years before the occurrence of clinically recognizable disease" (Kannel et al., 1961, p. 33). Not only the notion of risk factor, but this idea of the coronary prone *individual* retained particular significance in the Framingham-based understanding of cardiovascular disease predispositions ever since. This continued as more risk factors were identified that became more explicitly linked to "certain habits and traits" (Dawber & Kannel, 1966). Even in the later formulation of combined, multifactorial risk profiles, functions and models these remained based on the individual and individual behaviour in particular (Kannel et al., 1976). By the time the initially planned two decades of studying the causes of heart disease drew to a close, the study infrastructure consisted of an established methodological and substantive approach to cardiovascular disease. This infrastructure framed heart disease in terms of individual risks that could be studied through the prospective observation of randomized cohorts. At the same time, the infrastructure was strongly tied to a local community of participants.

Nevertheless, this infrastructure was not fully static, and its most significant reconfiguration was directly linked to its initial solidification. As the Framingham Study approached its scheduled end point in the late 1960s, most of its initial aims in terms of advancing scientific understanding of the causes of cardiovascular disease had been achieved. At the same time, the substantial expansion of research funding that had facilitated the start of the study shortly after the Second World War was increasingly put in question. This raised the question which value could be expected from continued funding of the study. The Framingham Heart Study may thus be understood as a kind of sentinel of a coming shift in research funding from a "social contract" to "collaborative assurance" including stricter controls on how research money was spent that David Guston (2000) locates in the 1970s and 1980s. As a result, there was considerable concern that new accountability criteria would result in termination of the Framingham Study (Patel, 2012). Eventually, both quiet and public lobbying contributed to a continuation of the study past its original 20 years, albeit with some significant extensions and recalibrations to this infrastructure.

To address concerns that all relevant questions had been answered, the Study expanded the range of questions to be addressed. Not least among this expansion were the recruitment of two further cohorts of children and (later) grandchildren of the original participants and their spouses in the Offspring (Feinleib et al., 1975) and Third Generation (Splansky et al., 2007) cohorts. Among other things, the recruitment of these cohorts allowed the study of familial and genetic aspects of cardiovascular disease, based on both the presence of biological relations (between parents and children) and their absence (to not biologically related spouses). In a sense, the idea of a randomized sample was thereby maintained in spite of the not-so random relations between the generations, as the unrelated spouses served as a kind of control group for genetic hypotheses.

To address concerns about accountability and productivity, the operation of the study was in some sense uncoupled from its coordination and management. While the "intramural" study clinic in Framingham continued to exist and be staffed with NHLBI employees, the study was formally transferred to Boston University (BU). The study has since been funded by the NHLBI on the basis of 7-year contracts with BU.[3] These contracts concern the 'core' of the study and describe BU's responsibilities for continued surveillance of cardiovascular events, exams of the study population and maintenance of the study clinic, data and sample collections etc. in a so-called Statement of Work. In addition, NHLBI and BU can agree to contracts for ancillary studies or supplementary work. The Framingham Study is required to report on the appropriate use of tax dollars to the Office of Management and Budget every 3 years. For each new contract period, the NHLBI proposes a list of "Initiatives" on the basis of recommendations from an external advisory committee. The Council of the NIH advises on these initiatives, but it is ultimately the NHLBI director who decides what goes into the new contract. Meanwhile, in Framingham the long established ethics advisory board that includes researchers, local political and religious authorities and residents continues to evaluate whether research plans are acceptable to the local community.

The particular institutional configuration forms an important part of the infrastructuring of cardiovascular disease research in the study. Governance and funding arrangements shape which kinds of work is possible in the study. The agreements between NIH and BU, for example, define quite clearly which kinds of work have to be done. Maintenance of the infrastructure itself is thereby defined as a significant task. This shows how the possible lines of research for the study are shaped not only by material aspects of methods, hypotheses and diagnostic criteria determined in the past, but also by organizational aspects. At the same time, organization also reflects particular imaginations of the study's place in the world. Here this takes the shape of solidifying ties to the local community via an advisory board including local luminaries. Yet the imaginative side of infrastructuring is also shaped through the separation of funding and operation, which reflects concern over accountability and the appropriate role of governmental institutions in scientific practice (see also Chap. 5).

Additionally, more widely changing configurations of medical research have also left their traces on the FHS. Particularly the growing scale and importance of collaborative networks in research have meant that Framingham is now more tightly interwoven with other research sites. One researcher explained to me how collaboration in itself is nothing new, but it had long been on a small scale, primarily with institutions in the region or with people further afield with whom personal contacts existed. At present, however, data and materials circulate much more widely, in part in response to the idea that larger data sets are required for research on the intricate (genetic) biology of common diseases such as heart disease (Davies et al., 2013). Another researcher described how, within the Framingham Study, it has been established practice to collect different kinds of samples—such as blood plasma, whole blood and cell lines—in order to be able to get as much diverse materials as possible and have them available for a long time. This person estimated that wider circulation of materials, collaboration and meta-analysis of existing studies can all contribute to advancing general insight into cardiovascular disease. This is in part achieved by the inclusion of all data from the FHS 'core studies' in the NIH Database of Genotypes and Phenotypes (dbGaP). At the same time, the highly touted community basis of the

Framingham Study figures in divergent ways in this context—both with regard to the accessibility of blood samples and data and in terms of the particular, family-based constitution of the Framingham cohorts. These are important aspects of both the imaginative dimensions of the Framingham research infrastructure and its practical affordances.

The Framingham Study as "A Beacon for the World"?

Beyond their functional role in allowing people, matter and ideas to circulate, infrastructures can also have symbolic and affective meanings (Larkin, 2013). The promise of infrastructure is part of its material configuration, both in how the ways infrastructures are built is based on more than just functional criteria and how the multi-layered history of an infrastructure can generate affect (Knox, 2017; Street, 2012). Affective connections to infrastructure can be local, but can also be attached to global circulations of (the idea of) a particular infrastructure. Thus, the idea of Framingham as a beacon to the world in this section's title refers to how the study may be an inspiration for studies of heart disease elsewhere (Greenberg, 2010). When I spoke to NHLBI staff over lunch during a visit to their offices, they similarly framed Framingham as the original epidemiological study of heart disease in the United States. They then went on to position the study as part of a broader 'portfolio' of epidemiological studies that collectively address the shortcomings of Framingham in terms of (especially) ethnic diversity. The idea of this portfolio, so NHLBI staff informed me, is to piece together different cohorts to something that kind of looks like a national biobank, which is allegedly difficult to establish in the United States due to the lack of a centralized, national health care system. Nevertheless, the various portfolio studies each have unique characteristics that make comparisons and continuities over time difficult.[4]

Indeed, the Framingham Heart Study has widely been critiqued for its reliance on an almost entirely white population. Yet, even though NHLBI staff presented the idea of a portfolio as an explicit effort to address a lack of diversity, analysts of the cultural intersections between heart disease and race in the United States have questioned this line of thinking. The Framingham Study continues to serve as a reference point for cardiovascular epidemiology (Shim, 2014). This implies that the particular approach to epidemiology developed in Framingham and extrapolation of its results continue to shape thinking about heart disease in the United States. Anne Pollock (2012), for example, compares the Framingham Study to the Jackson Heart Study, which focuses on a Black population. As Pollock shows, this study copied the idea of residential sampling from Framingham, while considering certain (social) risk factors relevant for its particular population that were seen as off-limits in Framingham. The Framingham Omni cohort, on the other hand, which was recruited in response to NIH diversity requirements, is too small to draw conclusions about any one specific group and maintains a residential rather than hereditary approach to its sample (Pollock, 2012). The Framingham Heart Study hence serves as a model for cardiovascular disease epidemiology in populations that are much more diverse than the original FHS cohort. At the same time, it continues exclusions considered irrelevant at the beginning, which are now reinforced by treating other study populations differently.

In spite of some of the Framingham Study's situated specificities, however, it is not only its design that has drawn interest from heart disease studies elsewhere. So has its data. As one NHLBI employee told me, the Framingham Study has long had the reputation of being unwilling to share its data "outside the Boston area", but this has changed. To a significant degree, this has been due to data sharing requirements. In this regard, the same person described the Framingham Study as a "vanguard study", picking up on its historical reputation to explain that the study was the first to make its data from Genome-Wide Association Studies (GWAS), a form of genetic research (Flint, 2013), available via the NIH platform dbGaP. NIH funded studies have been obliged to make their data available on this platform since 2007 and most of the Framingham core study data and some of the data from ancillary studies is available there. Data is uploaded after an embargo period and one Framingham researcher maintained that, although the easy availability has resulted in less direct requests for Framingham data, the platform has resulted in more of a "sharing culture". At the same time, data sharing is not unfiltered—this person referred to a study that intended to look at a link between genetics and education. Since there was no clear link to heart disease, and presumably also because of the sensitive nature of such research, Framingham researchers decided not to share materials in this case.

The refusal to collaborate in this case once more accentuates a highly salient aspect of the affective meaning attributed to the Framingham infrastructure by its researchers, which is its tie-in to the local community. The importance of the community's contribution as research participants is regularly professed by study staff. In interviews, I was regularly reminded of the close relations between the study and the town's inhabitants—including former inhabitants who continued to participate in the study. One researcher summarized the point by stating that the study had not only invested in taking the community context seriously, but that participants also felt invested in the study. Furthermore, the researchers I interviewed would refer to a multi-generational legacy and warm relations between researchers and participants that were contrasted to ideas of more transactional links elsewhere. In making these claims, researchers were also quick to point out what they saw as the implications of the mutual investment between the study and the community. On the one hand, they indicated to feel a sense of responsibility towards participants and the confidentiality of their data—even when this would sometimes cause obstacles for collaboration. They would also argue that there was a sense of local pride and commitment to the study, which one researcher explained in terms of the unlikely contribution of a predominantly working-class community to scientific research. At the same time, the characterization of Framingham as a blue-collar town was also used to explain why certain types of research related to socioeconomic 'risk factors' had not been possible.

On the other hand, the long-standing relations between the town and the study were also understood to make certain forms of research possible that might be more difficult elsewhere. This has both an epistemic-methodological dimension, to which we will return later, and a socio-ethical one. Particularly in the domain of genetic research, so researchers indicated, there is much wider consent in Framingham then there appears to be in the general population (see also Levy et al., 2010). This is particularly the case for the Third Generation Cohort, which was planned and recruited as a cohort for genetic research from the beginning. To emphasize the imagined legacy of the study's community basis, researchers would hold up one particular example in which participants' trust was apparently nearly lost. In 1999, a proposal to establish a company for monetarizing the value of the Framingham data—which one person described to me as "a dbGaP for profit" was met with severe local resistance. Since, as one person explained to me, the losses from withdrawal of study participants would probably be larger than the profits to be expected from the commercialization of existing data, the plan was eventually abandoned (Levy & Brink, 2005). Since there has been much ado (not least in the social sciences) about the potential commercialization and capitalization of the life sciences (Sunder Rajan, 2006; Cooper, 2008; Birch & Tyfield, 2013; Chiapetta & Birch, 2018), this particular episode in the history of the Framingham Study appears to be an anachronism. Yet it highlights once more the affective dimensions of this particular research infrastructure in which, to paraphrase interview respondents, there is a tension between being open to new research and being protective of participants—with concerns about participants often being considered quintessential to what makes the Framingham Study work.

Framingham in the Genomic Age and the Lasting Power of Infrastructure

Continued participation of the local community in the study has consistently been seen as a vital asset for the Framingham Study. However, the meaning of specific forms of collectivity in relation to infrastructures is subject to change over time (Collier et al., 2016). With the increasing importance of genetic research, an increasingly important dimension of the Framingham community has become the inclusion of multiple subsequent generations of *families* of participants.

The consideration of genetic factors within the Framingham Study has largely held pace with the expansion of genetic understandings of disease in medicine and medical research overall. Clustering of heart disease within families was seen early on in the study, and efforts to explain such clustering expanded from the 1970s onwards. Early findings on aggregations of disease and certain risk factors within families suggested there was a "strong genetic basis" (Myers & O'Donnell, 1999, p. 549) to certain factors, particularly where family histories of disease occurred that could not fully be explained by known (lifestyle) risks. Whereas some risk factors could be linked to a specific molecular basis, others could not—and the idea that specific genes for cardiovascular disease and risk factors could be found once DNA analysis developed from the late 1980s onwards (Govindaraju et al., 2008) largely did not bear out. Thus, the search for singular "candidate genes" was largely replaced by looking for associations between variants in the genome and disease outcomes in so-called Genome-Wide Association Studies (GWAS). For these studies the hope was that longitudinal phenotypical data on disease and risk factors from the multigenerational Framingham cohorts would allow the study to turn into a "gold standard [...] once again, this time in the genomic era" (Jaquish, 2007, p. 64). However, the hopes of GWAS were largely disappointed by the time I interviewed Framingham research staff in 2013, causing them to turn to a different argument for why this particular study was valuable for genomic research.

When I asked various Framingham Study researchers and administrators about the incorporation of genetic and genomic techniques in the study, they would point to the same advantage the study allegedly has. In the words of one researcher, this advantage consists of the availability of "sequential" data and samples from three generations of participants, many of whom are biologically related. This supposedly makes Framingham "a very different animal" from many other epidemiological studies, including those that have far large cohorts (across three generations, Framingham's totals less than 20,000).

After the aforementioned disappointments with GWAS, one researcher explained, geneticists came "full circle" and rediscovered the value of families for research on the genetics of cardiovascular disease. Another person who self-identified as a geneticist similarly highlighted the family structure as "quite powerful" for genetic research, while also emphasizing that genetic research requires good data on phenotypes. This person thus saw the potential of the Framingham Study for genetics in the presence of both families and longitudinal phenotypic data. In particular, these characteristics of the Framingham Study should allow the study of 'heritability' (i.e., to what degree can differences in disease occurrence be explained by genetics?) and clustering of cardiovascular disease and risk factors in families—rather than the identification of direct, Mendelian gene-disease links that appear to be exceedingly rare. Still another researcher explained the importance of families by arguing that the biological relations between people allow the study of genetics in a form not possible in a random sample of the same size. It allows one to trace genomic changes through multiple generations of a family and to link these to similar traces of disease incidence. Pointing in a similar direction, another colleague argued that it is possible to postulate a link between gene and risk factor in the first generation of participants, and then to see if the same link between genotype and phenotype can be found in the Offspring and Third Generation cohorts. This is supposed to give a more accurate picture of the significance of specific genetic variants. It also implies a re-interpretation of the study infrastructure in which there is a shift from the value of randomly selected participants to the value of not-so-random family relations.

While genetic research plays an increasingly important role among the study of various cardiovascular risk factors, this is not uncontroversial. One researcher recalled how, when the first initiatives towards genetic research emerged, many geneticists believed they would be able to 'really' make sense of disease, degrading epidemiologists to "phenotype collectors". Many epidemiologists, by contrast, remained sceptical of the promises of genetic research. They tended to think of genetics as one among various risk factors and one among many tools for epidemiology rather than the ultimate causal explanation. This tension is allegedly still not fully resolved—and, indeed, an epidemiologist I interviewed expressed concern that too much effort and resources were aimed at genomics. In his view, genetic associations can tell you whether there is a link between gene and disease or not, but does not explain the physiological and metabolic mechanisms of disease. To understand why things work as they do therefore requires other forms of research that consider more exposures than just genes.

My point in bringing up such disagreement is not to argue for one position or the other. Rather, I think it shows how even an established and by most accounts highly successful research infrastructure like the Framingham Study maintains a degree of interpretive flexibility (Bijker & Pinch, 1987). This flexibility of meanings attributed to the infrastructure here consists of the divergent interpretations of the relation between a multigenerational family-based cohort that is extensively phenotypically characterized as an asset for genetic research and the simultaneous view that an excessive focus on genetics contradicts the complex understanding of cardiovascular risks that has been generated from research on this same cohort.

This paradox of different interpretations also finds expression in the shifting meanings of materials kept within this infrastructure (cf. Radin, 2013). Shifts in meanings of stored materials result in part from technological developments as well as changing social and governance networks around tissue donation (Waldby & Mitchell, 2006). Catherine Waldby and Robert Mithcell further propose that the potential value of collected and stored tissues is shaped by the "technicity", or degree of technical manipulation of materials. However, approaching the collection of materials (primarily consisting of blood samples) in the context of the Framingham Study in terms of infrastructure further suggests that decisions made in the past continue to shape possibilities of manipulation and circulation. This is particularly the case in a study where the oldest samples still available date back to 1978, before large-scale and longitudinal use of these samples was of much interest to researchers.

When I visited the Framingham Study clinic, I also received a tour of the labs and storage facilities across the hall from the rooms where physical exams and blood collection take place. In 21 freezers there,[5] blood samples dating back to the late 1970s are kept for the study (with another 21 freezers located in the nearby town of Franklin). A lab staff member told me how 13 tubes of blood are taken at each examination, for a total of 101 ml. Most of this blood is stored in −80° freezers, with no immediate plans to use the samples. New samples are added to an already sizable collection. At the time, early in 2013, the lab had just made an estimate of the total number of samples stored—an exercise that took several months to complete and did not result in a more exact result than the observation that the number must have exceeded one million. The oldest samples stem from 1978 and include some participants from the first generation cohort—although those samples are often in a bad state. The storage is organized in boxes by exam cycle (e.g., Offspring Exam 9). Multiple samples from each individual are kept, in part because this allows investigation of changing blood values over time and in part because not all exams included the same analyses. Data kept about the samples as such included not only the examination cycle, but also a participant ID, the date the sample was taken, the box in which the sample is stored and its position within the box, as well as histories of sample shipping and use.

In line with aforementioned long-term effects of infrastructural design decisions made in the past, the person showing me the lab indicated that the samples "have lots of baggage" and that one would probably do things differently when starting a sample repository "from scratch". One example includes that the inventory of the freezers is kept in Excel and Access files (rather than more recent biological collection information systems), because it would be too much work to transfer them to other platforms.

Blood samples from the Framingham Study are not only stored in two sets of freezers in smaller cities in the state of Massachusetts. Some of the blood finds it ways to Boston University Medical Center. Blood is processed there in the Framingham genetics lab in order to actualize what Joanna Radin (2013) has described as the "latent life" of potential further use for new research purposes. In the BU lab, blood samples are processed to generate DNA, buffy coats, cell lines and other blood products that can be used for research. In addition, "forensic genotyping" is performed, an analysis of ten highly polymorphic markers that can be used to make sure a sample was actually taken from a specific donor.

The production of various blood products serves to maintain stock. Although individual research projects need far less than what can be generated from a single tube of blood, the supply is nevertheless limited. Samples at BU 'only' date back to the early 1990s, when genetic research started to become of serious interest to the Framingham Study. Cell lines have been produced since the late 1990s. The blood that is stored in various forms at BU is also available to other users—in fact, the processing at BU serves sample storage more than direct research uses—who can request samples from the repository. A lab administrator explained to me that they know from experience that most analyses require 2–5 mg of material, which is why requests for 20 mg are usually rejected.

When the BU lab (or similarly the lab in Framingham) does agree to make materials available, requesters receive samples from multiple cohorts, from a specific cohort or according to specific selection criteria. To make sure samples are efficiently and correctly withdrawn from storage, BU uses robotics. Once withdrawn, samples are frozen and shipped, often after the procedure has been discussed with the prospective recipient. One central requirement for sharing is that all data generated in the analysis is returned to the Framingham Study and, after an embargo period to allow publication, is also stored in dbGaP. This database provides access to complete datasets as it contains data on the individual level of research participants. The collection of blood samples from the study is thereby a functional infrastructure for cardiovascular disease research that can generate additional data for the study through sharing.

The blood samples collected over the course of the Framingham Study draw interest from researchers elsewhere for various reasons. The visibility of the study as a landmark epidemiological infrastructure is undoubtedly among them, as are the aforementioned advantages of the particular configuration of its study population. Yet it also reflects a wider desire to build larger study populations for genomic research. For Framingham Study researchers, on the other hand, a major advantage of sharing materials is that the study has generated too much data to be analysed in Framingham alone. Interestingly, the study as such is increasingly detached from the data and sample infrastructure it has generated in the process. This is both due to the organizational separation rooted in the contractual relations between BU and the NHLBI that I delved into above; at the same time, the storage of blood samples as a repository rather than for direct use also contributed to this status. In that sense, the Framingham Study can be thought of as "bigger" as an infrastructure than it is as a study. This observation aligns with Sabina Leonelli's (2013) analysis of the infrastructuring of contemporary 'big biology', yet she also observes how the relations between the global circulation and local production and adoption of data are characterized by frictions.

For Framingham researchers, these frictions are located between the desire of partners elsewhere to have fast and unfettered access to study materials, and (once more) restrictions legitimated in terms of concern for the Framingham community. In particular, there are certain uses of their blood—one researcher mentioned the reproductive use of cell lines—to which segments of the Framingham Study participants have not consented. This issue is not unique to the Framingham Study. The question how to balance potential new uses of available samples with respect for the donors' wishes forms perhaps one of the most hotly contested issues around the storage and use of blood and other bodily materials in medical research (Grande et al., 2014; Smilan, 2022). In the Framingham Study, this problem is addressed with a technical solution, which is described as tiered consent.[6] Perhaps unsurprisingly, the study leans towards prioritizing donor consent in sharing materials and will only release data of participants who have consented to a particular use of the materials. As one researcher summarized the procedure, the data of people who did not consent is excluded by data managers "at the door". This means their data is not sent out, and without associated data, samples are widely seen as useless for research.

Beyond such specific exclusions, the Framingham Study maintains a set of general criteria for when to make materials available or not. These include that the proposed use of the materials needs to be based on a clear hypothesis, that use of the materials needs to result in a publishable analysis and that the study for which the materials are used need to be related to cardiovascular outcomes.[7] However, the latter criterion appears to leave some room for interpretation. At the time of my visit to the Framingham clinic, materials had been shared with researchers focused on influenza. As a study staff member explained it, the influenza research group needed blood samples from multiple generations to see whether antibodies remaining from past episodes of the flu were reactivated with new infections (results from this study have been published in (Miller et al., 2013)). The link to the core remit of the Framingham Study in this case was found in the fact that mortality from influenza often happens through cardiovascular failure. In these and other cases, the blood samples that have been collected during the past four to five decades of the Framingham Study have thus come to be part of an infrastructure of research materials that builds on the pre-existing study infrastructures and the various lines of research it affords and restricts.

The continuity that—despite some occasional revisions—runs through the history of the Framingham Study and becomes especially visible when thinking through this research effort as an epidemiological infrastructure does not only concern the study's organizational coordinates, or central imaginaries of community and family. There is an equally strong epistemic continuity that reiterates the study's two key innovations of prospectively studying a randomly selected population and of introducing the idea of risk factors to medical research (Kannel & Wilson, 2007). Particularly the idea of the risk factor served as a key point of reference for Framingham Study researchers I interviewed about current developments in the study. Retrospectively, several of them narrated the emerging interest in genetics in terms of a deeper understanding of pathways of disease and a further disaggregation of the notion of 'risk factors', rather than in terms of the molecular 'blueprints' for disease that had long been central to thinking about the role of 'genes' in biology (cf. Keller, 2000). One researcher hypothesized that genetics research in the Framingham Study had always built on earlier work on risk factors. This person expressed the idea that the core idea in the study had always been to study how "genes act in concert with the environment"—although it would not have been formulated in these terms in the 1970s and 1980s. A colleague echoed this sentiment, arguing that the Framingham model had always been about interactions between genetics and environment and the totality of risk factors.

However, social science analyses of the politics of infrastructure should remind us that —to use Langdon Winner's (1986, p. 26) formulation—"the technological deck has been stacked" in favour of some interests over others. Like technologies such as bridges and tomato harvesting machines in Winner's essay, an epidemiological research infrastructure equally builds order towards particular understandings of disease. Although such order may be ambivalent and the Framingham results are far from uncontested, it does stack the deck towards individual, lifestyle-induced risks. In answering my questions about genetics in the Framingham Study, one of the aforementioned researchers illustrated this point by emphasizing how risk factors are modifiable and that behaviour can still be changed, even against a genetic background. Ideas about how to prevent heart disease thus tend to continue to move along the road long laid out in the Framingham Study.

Conclusion: The Multi-layered Infrastructuring of Epidemiological Research

In this chapter, I described the 'infrastructuring' of the Framingham Heart Study from its beginnings in the late 1940s to the present. I explored how this study became an *infrastructure* for the purpose of population-based medical research in terms of its organizational, material and epistemic dimensions in both a functional and symbolic sense. I first traced the infrastructuring process in the first two-plus decades of the study, which included joint organizational and epistemic calibration of the involvement of NIH, the pursuit of a particular method (a prospective, randomized cohort study), and the 'testing' of specific hypotheses that predominantly leaned towards understanding how individual 'habits' contributed to cardiovascular disease. While these early developments have had long lasting effects on how cardiovascular research is done—both in the Framingham Study and beyond—the infrastructure has not been static. The threat of termination in the late 1960s—ironically a proof of sorts of the infrastructure 'working' up to that point—resulted in a set of reforms. These again were simultaneously organizational and epistemic, generating new forms of accountability through the study's outsourcing from the NHLBI to Boston University, and new research directions through studies of subsequent generations. These reforms, too, have left traces on the Framingham Study infrastructure in the half century since.

The particular approach to studying cardiovascular disease that is at the centre of the study is also reflected in the affective significance it has attained both locally and globally. These affective dimensions have, in turn, shaped the forms of work the study affords. As a pioneering epidemiological study of heart disease, the study has obtained an influential reputation, in spite of its alleged reluctance to collaborate with researchers elsewhere. This reputation is at least in part due to an internal imaginary that the study is deeply rooted in and dependent on the local community (which also includes people who have moved away from Framingham, or are related to first generation residents). The perceived interests of this community hence shape many decisions, including those related to the ethics of data and sample sharing. It has particular implications for the use and sharing of blood samples, which, in the study's role as a repository, have taken on their own infrastructural form shaped by decades of collection, storage and use. Through a combination of Framingham Study organization, the materiality of storage and the (re-)emergence of a biological understanding of families, the growing focus on genomics in medical research has taken on a specific form in the Framingham Study. As an infrastructure for genomic research, it presents families as a highly valuable asset for studying genetic factors in association with other—still largely individual—risk factors. Looking at history and present of the Framingham Heart Study through an infrastructural lens thereby also shows how the 'social' and 'scientific' dimensions of medical research can never be fully separated. At its heart, the Framingham Study was made into a sociotechnical configuration foregrounding prospective searches for lifestyle-related, individual risk factors on a community—and in relation to genetics, family—basis.

This particular framing of disease risks that runs as a red thread through the work done in the context of the Framingham Study has far-reaching implications for the study's contributions to population health. The study has enabled certain—highly influential—measurements of risk, but also restricted and obscured others. This is one of the most consistently critiqued aspects of the study. On the basis of the Framingham Study, the notion of the risk factor has been developed such that it is mostly expressed in terms of individual behaviour (Giroux, 2013). Such a risk factor notion does not only restrict the understanding of the mechanics of disease, in spite of clear indications that social factors—including the social roots of lifestyle choices—play an important role in disease aetiology (Cockerham, 2013). The individualized risk factor simultaneously gives meaning to disease beyond the medical domain, framing heart disease risks in terms of individual responsibility and blame (Aronowitz, 1998; Bell, 2017).

Yet, the individualization of disease risks is just one example of how research infrastructures for studying cardiovascular disease—in all their complexity—frame to which populations particular understandings of disease apply, and how. The long-standing association between heart disease, (economic) wealth and modernity, for example, has long been expressed through a reading of heart disease as "White" and associated marginalization of other racial categories (Pollock, 2012).

Infrastructure can then be considered to shape social classifications around health and disease. As Janet Shim (2014, p. 4) writes:

> At multiple nodes of epidemiologic knowledge production—grant applications, data collection instruments, statistical software, and journal publications—and in multiple activities such as articulating research questions, collecting and analyzing data, interpreting results, and disseminating findings, epidemiology continually yet often imperceptibly legitimates particular definitions of race, class, and gender and systems for categorizing those differences.

Moving beyond individual studies, she thereby described how the organizational and epistemic dimensions of medical research intersect, rendering research infrastructures quintessentially sociotechnical. In turn, such infrastructures are intricately woven into categories of social classification, shaping how difference obtains meaning in medical research.

The classification and categorization of a population differentially affected by disease and the definition of particular mechanisms of disease should not be understood as the result of any actor's straightforward intention or bias. The continued consideration of racial differences in the context of heart disease, for example, is largely a product of race being available as a ready-made system of social classification. Race will therefore, so Anne Pollock (2012) writes, retain its medical significance as long as it continues to be used as a social category. Although by no means limited to the United States—and notwithstanding the global spread of racial framings of disease as a product of the far-reaching influence of US science across national borders—"racial" classifications of health and disease may look quite differently elsewhere (Felt et al., 2017; Kowal, 2022). Yet, racialized understandings of cardiovascular disease, as well as the restrictive individual notion of the risk factor, are the lasting effects of the particular environment in which a research infrastructure got made. This includes the uncertainties and disagreements that needed to be negotiated at the very beginning of the Framingham Study (Oppenheimer, 2005). The infrastructuring of medical research thus unavoidably implies the infrastructuring of its object—the disease, how it works, and whom it affects along pre-existing social as much as biological categories.

The history of the Framingham Heart Study indicates how an infrastructure for epidemiological research on cardiovascular disease was built. Zooming in on the present shows how this history and the particular configuration of the infrastructure shapes current research, both with a focus on genetic factors in cardiovascular disease and with regard to the study's function as a multigenerational, longitudinal repository. In both cases, decisions of the past have had lasting influence. The Framingham Study infrastructure that developed a risk factor notion focused on individual lifestyle and imagined itself deeply rooted in the community shaped the possibilities and obstacles for genetic research as well as which materials are available to be shared and how they can be circulated. This infrastructure simultaneously enables the performance of particular kinds of work and entails particular visions of how cardiovascular epidemiology should operate. It is also multi-layered and sociotechnical, combining, among others, institutions that fund, govern and operate the study, particular research methods, the community of participants and a vast collection of data and materials. All of these layers are woven together to build an infrastructure that shapes research in a particular way. Yet across these layers, different research purposes may be pursued, which is a dimension we look into in more detail in the next chapter.

Notes

1. The use of this particular metaphor to qualify Framingham as "average American town" is somewhat ironic. Its reference to diet suggests high local prevalence of certain risk factors, but due to the uniformity of local food consumption, the Framingham Study has not been able to definitively establish a link between diet and cardiovascular disease risks (Kannel & Wilson, 2007; Schiffman, 1970).
2. See (Dawber, 1980, p. 33) for a full list.
3. The following reconstruction of the current funding and governance of the study is based on interviews with NIH officials.
4. A particular dilemma with regard to the Framingham Heart Study appears to be that it is often slow to implement new approaches and measure-

ments, since they make comparison over time and thus the identification of continuity and change in cardiovascular disease rates difficult.

5. This was the case in 2013. The number of freezers would logically be larger now, unless some of the older samples have been discarded.
6. For a discussion of various alternative models to "specific" informed consent, see (Wiertz & Boldt, 2022).
7. For the formal Framingham data sharing principles, see https://www.framinghamheartstudy.org/fhs-for-researchers/policies-and-procedures/data-sharing-principles/ (last accessed 9 July 2025).

3

Contesting Research Collection Purposes in the Singapore Tissue Network

In the Spring of 2013, I was in Singapore to study what had caused the termination of the country's centralized biomedical research repository, when I was invited to join a staff meeting at one of the remaining institution-based repositories in one of Singapore's larger hospitals. In this meeting, I joined the head of the repository and eight staff members—many of whom, it turned out in a conversation afterwards, had come to Singapore from elsewhere in Southeast Asia—to discuss the collection and withdrawal of tissue samples. Guiding us through the state of the repository was a set of PowerPoint slides, full of tables and charts that showed for different (tumour) tissues how much had been collected, requested for research, withdrawn from the repository and ultimately used for scientific publications during specific time periods. And so I learned, for example, that there had been 146 cases of 'unscheduled' collection in January, and 83 in February, with most of the tissue originating from patients' colons. While showing the slides, the head of the repository made a point of arguing for unscheduled collection—which means that a sample is taken without immediate plans for use in a specific research project—since, he explained, in those cases any researcher could use the sample at some point. He further observed how, with limited staff, he preferred more focus on collecting breast cancer tissue—a focal

E. Aarden, *Producing Citizenship in Medical Research Collections*, Health, Technology and Society, https://doi.org/10.1007/978-981-95-1707-7_3

research area in the hospital—at the expense of colon tissue, of which he believed to have enough. Although it was not described in these terms, the meeting thus revolved around how specific *purposes* of a tissue repository manifested in tissue collection practices as well as the collection itself.[1]

The meeting's focus on which specific forms of tissue to collect and why, which included considerations of research priorities and likelihood of publication, covers just some of the possible purposes that can be ascribed to collections of tissues and data. Particularly around the early twenty-first century 'boom' of national biobanking projects (Kaiser, 2002), tissue and data collections became associated with (often unspecified) scientific, medical, but also economic, political and broader national cultural intentions (Winickoff, 2006; Busby & Martin, 2006; Benjamin, 2009). A key aspect of this wave of initiatives were wide-ranging promises of progress associated with the "potentiality" of tissue materials to obtain as-yet unknown uses and generate as-yet unknown benefits (Taussig et al., 2013). The Singaporean government's decision to include a centralized tissue repository called Singapore Tissue Network (STN) in its investments in building up a biomedical research and industry sector around the turn of the century can be considered one example of initiatives that simultaneously took place in places as diverse as Iceland, the United Kingdom, Estonia, China and many more (see, e.g., Gottweis & Petersen, 2008; Sleeboom-Faulkner, 2009).

However, the rather brief biography of Singapore's centralized repository, which started as STN in 2003 and was called Singapore Biobank (SBB) by the time it closed in 2011,[2] shows how the multiple purposes attributed to biobanking projects do not necessarily align. In particular, the persistence of institution-based repositories in the aftermath of STN/SBB's closing suggests that researchers continued to see a purpose for tissue repositories, even if the government's funding agencies no longer did—at least at a centralized national scale. In this chapter, I therefore delve into the fate of what I will from now on mainly describe as the Singapore Tissue Network as well as Singapore's remaining tissue repositories. I will explore different understandings of their purposes and how these informed design and operations. I first draw on work in STS that discusses imaginations, expectations and promises of different forms of scientific, economic, social and other value to trace how purposes for biobanking in Singapore were formulated. I will show how these tied into the specific positioning of biomedical research as a historically situated economic development effort in Singapore, as well as into the promissory dynamics of biobanking vis-à-vis both notions of an emerging 'bioeconomy' and the economy of credibility and recognition in science.

In a next step, I link these imaginations to the practical operations of tissue repositories. I start from the idea that the value of a repository or of the materials it contains is not given, but rather gets produced in practices of donor recruitment, tissue collection, processing and storage—including procedures of caring for tissue and data quality—as well as retrieval and use. A key aspect of such value creation is that it ties specifics of biomedical research in Singapore to broader concerns in the medical research field that appear to emerge largely independent of specific locations. Nevertheless, the specific characteristics of Singapore ultimately matter in the closing of the STN—which thereby presents a particularly interesting case for looking into the tensions that may occur between different purposes of a biobank. I will consider such tensions in the final section of the chapter and again link these to broader concerns around the proclaimed importance of data circulation in biomedical research.

Imagining Purposes of Biomedical Research Repositories

The Singapore Tissue Network was established as a centralized repository for human tissues collected for biomedical research in different research projects. It thereby served, to quote one policy official, as a 'support structure' for research. It distinguished itself from some centralized national biobanks elsewhere by not collecting any tissue itself. As this same person explained, the centralized repository was expected to contribute to so-called "translational" research linking laboratory findings to clinical applications (see, e.g., Murtagh et al., 2011). He argued that "in order to do good translational research, you needed tissues (...) and [in Singapore] it was thought it should be centralized, because then everyone could have access". Pursuing similar arguments, other interview respondents pointed to STN as a centralized storage facility that generated specific advantages for biomedical research in Singapore, especially with regard to reducing the overall costs of tissue storage and the ability to "...profit from the compactness of Singapore and economies of scale, that it is easy to skip things around". Focusing on such "economies of scale", STN was thus primarily aimed at high quality storage and much less at how materials might eventually be used.

In those early years of the present century, Singapore was far from the only country establishing a centralized tissue repository or biobank. In the words of an administrator working for the network at the time, "it was a bit of a trend that countries were setting up national tissue repositories". Many of such repositories, so Aaro Tupasela (2017b) has observed, presented (national) populations "as brands". Such branding turns a population into "a type of product whose unique characteristics are designed to attract scientific and commercial interest" (Tupasela, 2017b, p. 2). Branding of a population is furthermore linked to particular "imaginaries" of a scientific, medical and sociopolitical context in which research on such a branded population may thrive. Nordic European countries are widely discussed as exemplars of sites that are promoted as especially promising for population research (see also Chap. 5), which is often framed in terms of the supposed relative biological homogeneity of the population, the presence of continuous long-term population health data (often linked to material samples) and a close relation to the welfare state as both a source of research participation and a readily available market for applications (Cool, 2016; Tupasela et al., 2020). At the same time, the large scale collection and use of samples and materials for medical research are often linked to future economic competitiveness and cost reductions in health care. As Kadri Simm (2010) has observed for the national biobank in Estonia, national biobank projects often serve to simultaneously legitimate biomedical research as a worthy domain of public investment and the state as a key actor in economic growth and innovation.

The various ways medical research repositories get linked to economic growth, progress in healthcare and the continued contemporary viability of the nation state point to the key role of promises and expectations in national biobanking projects. Herbert Gottweis and Alan Petersen (2008) have therefore described expectations surrounding biobanks, as well as the rhetoric of nation-building and the economic promise of research and innovation in biotechnology as key issues in biobank governance. Exploring similar ideas, Mike Fortun (2008) has described promises as an essential aspect of the establishment of the Icelandic Health Sector Database, a widely discussed example of a national biobanking project. Yet research on promises and expectations in other domains of technological innovation has demonstrated how promises can turn into requirements for developers to indeed produce the anticipated outcomes (Borup et al., 2006; Van Lente, 2000). In biobanking, expectations thus have effects on the meanings attributed to tissue collections and how they are operated (Tarkkala, 2019). One researcher in Singapore thus described how “the idea [of a centralized tissue repository] was that people would share [materials] and industry would like it”. This idea was integrated into the repository’s design, but turned out much more challenging to actualize in biobanking operations.

My interview respondent’s reference to industry, however, illustrates the main reasoning behind the establishment of a national tissue repository in Singapore. The STN can be seen as an integral part of the ‘infrastructure’ for biomedical research that was built up in the context of the Biomedical Sciences Initiative (BMSI) launched by the Singapore government in 2000. The idea of this initiative, according to one policy official, was to “jumpstart biomedical research with economic objectives”, and thus to invest not in “science for its own sake, but to create more jobs in Singapore”. In contrast to the aforementioned cases in Nordic Europe, a national biobank in Singapore was thus not linked to a notion of a welfare state—which is generally a suspect notion there (see Lim, 2010)—but to ideas of medical excellence and of establishing a novel area of economic activity.

The BMSI may therefore be understood as a continuation of an established ‘developmentalist’ agenda in which national governments explicitly seek to push economic development in specific sectors (see, e.g., Schein, 1996; Wong, 2011; Yew, 2011). Along these lines, a senior policy official characterized the BMSI as “a big decision by the government after watching what was going on in the rest of the world. So, in Singapore we always look what we can do five or ten years down the road”. This big decision, he continued, involved the identification of biomedical research as an area with great economic potential. His description of the initiative thereby flags various aspects that have been characterized as key dimensions of Singapore's economic growth agenda since the country gained independence in the 1960s.[3] These include the explicit reliance on foreign investment, experience and expertise, along with long-term development plans for specific sectors. This strategy has further involved a shift from production to research and development in ever-more advanced technological sectors as prioritized sectors of the economy (Lee, 2008; Gelfert, 2013). This trend supposedly culminated in an "emerging emphasis on high tech startups and the shift towards technology creating capabilities" (Lee, 2007, p. 167) since the late 1990s.

Yet even though investments in biomedical research appear to form a continuation of a policy tradition often captured with the Singapore Inc. moniker,[4] the shift towards research entailed some discontinuities with earlier economic development efforts. Rather than only attracting foreign investment and expertise, biomedical research—largely focused on genomics in the early twenty-first century—tied Singapore into particular global scientific networks (Thacker, 2005). This affected how the country is positioned both within Asia and beyond. At the same time, biomedical research forms a discontinuity with earlier brandings of Singapore that moved away from the material, and certainly from anything having to do with disease (Clancey, 2012). In that sense, Clancey argues, the BMSI not only reflects a particular tradition of economic development and national branding in Singapore, but also a particular moment in time characterized by an increasing emphasis on globally connected cities and an understanding of the genome as code. Singapore's decision to focus on biomedical research thereby reflects particular imaginations of the country's place in the world and the role of science and technology in its global advancement.

Literature in science and technology studies (STS) has described these kinds of national political designs to be realized through or with science and technology as sociotechnical imaginaries (Jasanoff & Kim, 2009, 2015; McNeil et al., 2017). This notion aims to convey the idea that science and technology do not only have material effects in the world, but may also be incorporated into particular views of what a nation, or any other human collective is and can and should aspire to be. In relation to Singapore, the idea that imagination has had a core function in making the nation is widespread (Lim, 2002; Ban et al., 2004; Yao, 2007). It is also visible in the throughlines drawn between early industrialization and the present investments in biomedical research.[5]

While this idea of sociotechnical imaginaries makes the role of science and technology in nation-building and the associated sociopolitical intentions of investments in research and innovation explicit, work in this vein often has little to say about scientific practice. Considering the wide range of purposes associated with biobanking, and biomedical research at large in Singapore—not all of which directly fit the state's agenda—we may additionally draw on George Marcus' (1995) contrasting notion of technoscientific imaginaries. This notion considers how socially and culturally situated imaginaries shape scientific practice. The technoscientific imaginary "indeed looks to the future and future possibility through technoscientific innovation but is equally constrained by the very present conditions of scientific work" (Marcus, 1995, p. 4). Jointly, sociotechnical and technoscientific imaginaries can draw our analytical attention to both the ways science and technology are mobilized for sociopolitical purposes and how such purposes may shape, but also be challenged by, the purposes of scientific work. As such, an analytical focus on imaginaries may help explore the various answers to the question why science is done or, more specifically, why human tissue and data are collected and stored.

Imagining the future has clearly been a central element in Singapore's investments in biomedical research, but not without some reservations. Both social science analyses of and commentaries in scientific journals on the BMSI have questioned the implications of the explicitly economic imaginaries attached to biomedical research in Singapore. Particularly in the first decade of the initiative influential scientific journals such as *Science* and *Nature* expressed occasional discomfort with ongoing developments. They often combined celebrations of the considerable financial investments in science with concern over the role of an authoritarian government and the country's supposedly immature scientific culture (Swinbanks, 1999; Cyranoski, 2001; Smaglik, 2003; Birmingham, 2001; Normile, 2007, 2011). Similarly, yet from a slightly different angle, social science critics questioned Singapore's biomedical research endeavours as a continuation of its "constitutive utopian vision in the mode of biological innovation" (Waldby, 2009b, p. 371). Such critics emphasize the outward looking character of biomedicine in Singapore, arguing that its aim to tie into global research and innovation networks happens at the expense of the local population. This population is supposedly turned into experimental subjects not otherwise actively engaged in building research capacities in Singapore (Waldby, 2009a, b; Holden & Demeritt, 2008).

Parallel to such concerns about the implications of the BMSI for the local population, other commentators have focused on the role of high-profile foreign scientists recruited to lead institutions in Singapore. They relate such recruitments as well as the country's positioning in global networks to how Singapore has sought to advertise its relevance for global biomedical research with reference to Asia—both in logistical terms of providing a gateway to large Asian markets for pharmaceutical and biotechnology companies, and in biological terms as a location where major Asian populations can be found at a relatively concentrated scale (Kuo, 2012). These observers highlight how the global and economic significance of biomedical research in Singapore is mediated through its Asian location and character (Ong, 2013; Fischer, 2013). Aihwa Ong in particular has unfolded the significance of Singapore as a stand-in for Asia in biomedical research. She discusses various forms of such Asian representativeness—ranging from the reification of colonial racial categories that present the country as "a scalable genetic microcosm of the vast continent's population" (Ong, 2015, p. 333) to more nebulous anxieties about national identity and prestige informing biotechnology efforts across Southeast Asia (Ong & Chen, 2010).

In spite of such arguments that (to different degrees) detach biomedical research in Singapore from its population and place it at a regional or global level, a closer look at specific institutional formations such as a national tissue repository suggests different insights. In this regard, I draw on Charis Thompson's (2010, p. 122) work on stem cell research in Singapore and South Korea and her observation that "what it is to have been an Asian Tiger and now be participating in the age of biotechnology is a heterogeneous affair". Both the specifics of the "baroque ecology" of

Singapore's Biopolis research campus (Ong, 2006b, p. 180) as well as specific aspects of how Singapore does biomedical research matter. For example, one government official succinctly summarized specific advantages he saw for Singapore, referring in an interview to "Western-style" medicine practised in the country and the widespread use of English.

How these alleged advantages are supposed to manifest in practice can, for example, be seen in reflections on the role of the Bioethics Advisory Commission (BAC) that was established in the context of Singapore's biomedical research investments. In an edited volume on the BAC's work, its role in attuning research in Singapore to international networks and their criteria for 'good science' is made quite explicit (Ho & Lim, 2010). This does not mean, however, that bioethics is considered an exclusively foreign input in the research landscape. Rather, BAC recommendations are framed as "uniquely Singapore in their pragmatism, looking for solutions rather than positions" that take both international views and local context into account (Chan & Liu, 2010, p. 42). Moreover, I observed in various conversations, at public forum discussions on biomedical research and in local newspapers how particular local concerns were never far away in the design, practices and purposes of biomedical research in Singapore. These ranged from the purportedly distinctly bureaucratic management of research institutions to the challenges posed by an ageing population and other social transformations. Such examples indicate how Singapore was imagined vis-à-vis a global medical research environment.

Various aspects of the concerns, traditions and routines that inform biomedical research in Singapore can also be traced in the design and operations of the Singapore Tissue Network and successive tissue repositories. As a researcher described it in an interview, STN was conceived as a national tissue bank to be located at the Biopolis research campus. Since this location had the disadvantage of being removed from the hospitals where tissues would be collected,[6] the STN was established with various incentives for the hospitals. The most important one was the availability of free storage in the repository. In addition, a former STN employee explained, sample storage was supported to the extent that researchers "only had to provide the nurses for consent". Among the services STN supplied were dedicated sample kits, heat-resistant containers for transportation and a pick-up service for bringing the samples to Biopolis. Within one of the buildings at Biopolis, the STN was established as a largely automated biobank, with robots for moving samples around and only a limited number of staff. All this was done with the aim of storing samples in a standardized, sustainable and high-quality storage facility at lower aggregate costs than if samples would remain stored at the various institutions of projects' principal investigators.

While one researcher described it as self-evident that he stored sample with STN since "a bona fide researcher puts it where it is best stored", this sentiment was not shared by all researchers in Singapore. To nevertheless expand the storage of samples in the Tissue Network, several changes to the repository's set-up were made early on. One was to require all recipients of national research grants to store any samples they collected in the centralized repository, while simultaneously not providing funding for tissue storage elsewhere. Another reform was for STN to no longer maintain full control over stored materials. Instead, the network introduced a so-called 50–50 rule, which implied that whoever contributed a sample maintained exclusive access to half of the sample, while the other half would be accessible to researchers via the STN access procedure. A former STN employee described this arrangement as "a fair exchange" where "in order not to have to pay to store your tissue, you have to give up half of it".

At the same time, he described STN as "custodian of the samples, not owner". Although it would be the network's steering committee that would decide on who got access to samples or not, the network itself held only limited descriptive data on those materials. This was done deliberately; since in-depth data on the samples is required to be able to use them in research, research funding agency A*STAR' imagined that the need to contact the person who had placed a sample in the repository for clinical data would lead to novel collaborations between sample users and suppliers. The fact that this did not happen to the anticipated degree was a major factor in the STN shutting down; to understand *why* this happened it is helpful to delve deeper into the purposes researchers attribute to sample collections and how these inform the ways they work with samples from the recruitment of donors until and including the use of samples in research and for scientific publications.

Tissue Practices and the Purposes of Collection

The establishment of a centralized tissue repository in the context of an economic strategy rooted in research and innovation in the life sciences may be seen in a broader context. As mentioned above, similar institutions were established around the globe around the same time. Even where these biobanks less assertively pursued an economic agenda, imaginaries of (future) profits from stored tissues circulated widely. The materials stored in biobanks can thereby be considered to be "assets" in the register of technoscientific capitalism: imbued with imagined future value that legitimates investments in the present (Birch & Muniesa, 2020). Yet biomaterials are not only valued as economic assets, nor is this particular valuation given in advance. As Dussauge and co-authors (2015c, p. 1) write, "[t]he social and material orderings of the life sciences and health care are permeated with the making, attribution and performance of different values: cultural, economic, legal". Different forms of value(s), they maintain, are enacted in practices. Values should therefore "be seen as always already constituted in practices, not as static entities which exist outside of action" (Dussauge et al., 2015c, p. 19). When considering the (often anticipatory, as-yet unrealized) values attributed to tissue and data collections (and thus, I would say, the purposes for which these materials were collected), we may therefore think in terms of different "spheres" of value aligned with distinct expectations, possible applications as well as institutional formations pursuing distinct kinds of "value" (Burton et al., 2021).

Focusing on the "making of" of different kinds of value in tissue repository practices shows how this is not merely a matter of extracting value that is already latently there through the technical manipulation of biological materials (Waldby & Mitchell, 2006; Chiapetta & Birch, 2018). Rather, generating different forms of value is the product of a combination of biological materials themselves, the practices in which materials are processed and institutional design and operations of repositories as well as research institutions through which the materials circulate. In other words, value generation in biobanking continuously takes place along the entire 'lifespan' of samples and data ranging from donor recruitment through their collection, processing and storage, up to moments of retrieval, sharing and use (Aarden, 2024). With a focus on data that can equally be applied to tissue samples, Tahani Nadim (2016) thus speaks of data labour. This includes "the routine tasks that tend to data: cleaning, managing, organizing, storing data so that they can be found, searched and used" (Nadim, 2016, p. 498). Such practices of caring for data (and tissues) "represent an important mechanism of value creation for the laboratory" (Pinel et al., 2020, p. 178).

Yet value here, again, does not only refer to economic value, but also includes the "affective, attentive and relational dimensions of data work" (Pinel et al., 2020, p. 179). Hence, a wide range of values may be produced through and attributed to stored research materials at different moments of practical engagement with the data. At the same time, (expected) value creation is not only a hands-on practical achievement, but also involves an adjustment of institutional arrangements to the forms of value pursued. Focusing on "translational" eye research in Singapore, for example, Cathelijne Coopmans et al. (2012) traced how this purpose can be achieved by extending existing research trajectories and making the clinic more like a research facility. Not only the work done in biobanks, but also how a biobank is organizationally configured contributes to how specific kinds of value(s) can(not) be generated.

With this multiplicity of values and of value-creation practices in mind, it is useful to look in more detail at the way repositories in Singapore work (or worked). As a starting point, it is worth noting how, in contrast to some (but not all) 'national' biobanks elsewhere, STN did not collect materials itself. There was thus no national donor recruitment programme and, indeed, various interview respondents highlighted how STN was located at the Biopolis research campus, a place without hospitals where donors could be recruited. Recruitment was left to clinicians or researchers who ran individual research projects, who could decide under which criteria to recruit. This also meant that STN, overall, did not aim for any specific characteristics (e.g., representativeness) in its collection, even though the BMSI as a whole strongly emphasized the 'Asian' character of Singapore's population.

In the recruitment of tissue donors for research projects, we encounter a rather broad but important distinction in the types of tissues collected for research repositories. For so-called solid tissues such as samples taken from tumours, the donors commonly are already committed to the hospital for surgery. Asking for their consent to store (parts of) a tumour after it has been surgically removed, so staff members of a tumour tissue repository assured me, is relatively straightforward. Asking after surgery is allegedly "the proper thing to do" since it avoids further stress for the patient prior to their operation. Only if tissue is not frozen but used 'fresh' (e.g., for creating cell lines) should consent be obtained pre-surgery. This is different from collecting so-called liquid tissue, which mainly involves blood samples as well as other bodily fluids such as urine and saliva. Liquid samples are often (but not always) collected in cohort studies for which potential participants have been selected and invited to participate voluntarily and independently of any healthcare encounters. For such sampling, the selection and recruitment process is often more complex.

In the previous chapter, I discussed how the Framingham Study early on introduced the idea of random selection of participants, which has since become an epidemiological gold standard. In interviews about the recruitment for epidemiological studies, researchers in Singapore would sketch a similar scenario. One study director, for example, explained how for his study, he had used Singapore's electoral register to start and invite randomly selected candidates for participation, beginning with people living in the vicinity of the clinic. Yet such recruitment is not entirely random; in line with the emphasis on Singapore as a microcosm for Asia, many studies focus on one of the 'traditionally' recognized ethnic groups of Chinese, Malays and Indians. This distinction has considerable administrative relevance in Singapore and is also used for structuring recruitment in research, even if it is less clear that biologically or medically relevant differences between these groups can actually be found (Coopmans & Tan, 2018). One research institute where I did interviews on recruitment and data and tissue collection in cohort studies ran different studies for each of the three main ethnic groups. For each of these studies, potential participants first received an invitation letter, followed by a phone call and eventually a couple of home visits. In total, I was told, four efforts to get a person to participate would be made.

A study coordinator explained how recruitment was often a complex and time-consuming process that got progressively more difficult as people were requested for follow-up studies. Recruitment also seemed to be shaped by various considerations of how to best account for particularities of (social) life in Singapore. In many cases, individuals would supposedly come to the clinic to complain or receive study incentives, without the intention of participating in the study. Since this research institute primarily did research on elderly people, further complexities arose from getting study participants to come to the clinic—for which either recruiters' organized transportation or examinations were scheduled on Saturdays, so that family members could come with the study participants. Study coordinators and clinical staff also delivered a kind of social services for participants, often caring for those that seemed undernourished or dehydrated. In case anything suspicious was found during examinations, people got a follow-up appointment at the clinic for further care. The recruiters who visited potential participants at home were also the ones who went through the questionnaires with people who do participate, in order to "make sure they see a familiar face". These recruiters were also "ethnically matched" to the people they recruited, again to create a sense of familiarity and trust. Through these recruitment practices, study participants were thus treated as more than just research objects—even if obtaining their blood and data remained the ultimate goal. In the recruitment and examination context, (potential) research participants were thereby framed in terms of their ethnicity and in relation to specific concerns clinic staff have with regard to social relations in Singapore.

People recruited for studies at this particular institute are asked to contribute data and tissue to medical research. Data was gathered with questionnaires and clinical examinations. Since some of the studies have been quite successful in recruitment and productive in publications, other researchers want to attach their research to these particular cohorts, resulting in a steady growth of the number of questionnaires to be filled out and measures to be taken. According to one recruiter, this requires further coordination in order not to make participation too exhausting. The collection of tissue here takes the form of drawing a blood sample. Researchers insisted in interviews that tissue samples (or what they described as "biomaterials") were important since "studies with biomaterials last longer and have better, more robust findings". They do, for example, allow measurements to identify medical conditions the donor may not have been aware of. In addition, "the reason for collecting all these samples is that, in the future, there may be new questions. That's the basic reason for a biobank". Generating a blood sample is thus considered important for enhancing the (future) value of a study cohort. Yet it is not always easy, a coordinator explained. Especially older people are said to be "a bit resistant". The solution then is to "tell them it is good to have [some medical exams] and taking blood for biochemistry and, since it's the same needle, we take a bit more for future generations. And they buy it". As this example illustrates, the future promise of sample collection is also used to promote participation.

Not only is the recruitment procedure different for the collection of solid tissue, it also requires a different approach to the collection of the materials themselves. This is both an effect of the particular material form of solid tissue samples and of their source. Tumour tissue needs to be collected and processed relatively soon after it has been removed from a person's body, needs to be carefully documented and should not interfere with either the surgery itself or with diagnosing a patient's condition. As staff members of one of Singapore's remaining tissue repositories explained, they ought to be informed if any surgery on a tumour of potential interest is taking place. Staff members of the repository would then wait in the sluice room just outside the operating theatre to be able to move in quickly once the tumour has been removed. According to the repository's director, collection of a tumour sample, including photographic documentation of its location of origin in the body, should be completed within less than 20 minutes. Only tumours with a diameter of more than two centimetres are taken and the person collecting the sample has to have pathology training. For this reason, the repository mostly employs (cheaper) staff from the lower wage countries surrounding Singapore.

Quality assurance is considered critical for storing samples, and any tumour sample is therefore cut into alternating slices for storage and quality control. Detailed description of the relative amounts of tumour, healthy tissue and necrosis in each slice are documented, as well as data on a specimen's history, including warm and cold ischemia time (referring to how long a sample has been disconnected from blood circulation), the time between harvesting and storage in liquid nitrogen and how long a sample has been stored. Part of the sample needs to remain available in case it is required for diagnostic purposes at a later stage. Samples are therefore not made available to researchers until 1 month after they have been collected.

Tissue repositories cannot be (too) selective with regard to which samples are collected. Like in the staff meeting I opened this chapter with, the same tissue repository director explained in an interview that "there is a simple reason" why, as far as possible all tumours are collected. He explained this with the example of retinoblastoma, which "is a rare tumour. If I start collecting when I have a request, it may take twenty years [to collect enough samples for a study]. So, to facilitate research, a biobank must collect all tumours". Since one never knows if these will ever be used, however, biobanks have high costs that are difficult to recoup from, for example, user fees. As this same director somewhat dramatically illustrated, if only one out of every 100 specimen is ever withdrawn, "who is going to pay for the 99 others?" This question illustrates the issue of biobanks' financial sustainability (see also Watson et al., 2014; Doucet et al., 2017), which plagued both the STN and its successor repositories.

While one interview respondent summarized the differences by saying that liquid tissue is easier to store since it does not degrade to the same degree and takes up less space, the maintenance of either kind of tissue as well as of any associated data requires a significant amount of work. I have described the processes required to prepare solid tissue for storage. Blood samples are often also not only kept whole, but also processed into components such as DNA, plasma or buffy coats (a layer between red blood cells and plasma that remains after centrifuging). In addition to all of the sample history data discussed above, the data manager of a research institute also mentioned that it is important to keep track of where all the samples are at any point in time. This turned out to be particularly challenging when STN closed and its contents were (supposedly) returned to whomever had contributed the materials. In some cases, however, this was not possible. In this regard, a researcher referred to "legacy issues" in cohort studies, by which he meant a discrepancy between principal investigators' plans to collect blood samples and follow up on the donors for, say, 25 years and the much more restricted availability of funding.

In the STN, storage was free of charge, and thus "they collect and store thousands of samples. After five years, the PI has no more funding and they are supposed to be kept for twenty-five years. That is not sustainable". Again, financial sustainability is highlighted, this time with direct reference to the difficulties surrounding STN. After this national network closed, managers of remaining repositories therefore invested much time and energy in developing financing models—in spite of an alleged lack of understanding of biobanking costs among researchers. A manager of a biobank that took in many of the STN's (blood) samples described how he reduced storage costs by moving the repository away from Biopolis and by letting go of much of the staff. At the same time, he highlighted various forms of accreditation he pursued to make the quality of his repository visible and recognizable.

The technical and organizational processes of storing and maintaining tissue and data collections discussed in interviews also require forms of data (and sample) labour and care discussed in the STS literature. Such work is also required to make stored materials usable for other researchers. Materials may be made more widely available through direct engagement with and attachment to samples and data. In these processes, materials are also imbued with distinct meanings and tied to imagined futures (Pinel & Svendsen, 2021). Researchers value their collections because of the way they increase the value of their studies as well as their own currency in the reputational economy of science (Latour & Woolgar, 1986). Researchers at one research institute would for example explain how, over time, interest in their data set had grown since there was ever more data to work with. Over time, they had arrived in a situation where "people now know [our] Singapore cohort better. Singapore is now more on the map". Yet, they maintained that this was not only a matter of the quality of the materials as such. One senior researcher additionally contended that "for science to progress, you need as much heroes and faces as hard science" This statement succinctly illustrates how the value of research materials is in part attached to and enhanced by their relations to particular persons or institutions.

These attachments also implied that collections may "belong to" or at least be associated with particular persons. This affects if, how, and when materials get shared. Sharing or circulation of materials is considered key to contemporary biological research and is associated "with massive efforts devoted to building infrastructures (databases, repositories, biobanks) for the dissemination of data across research locations, disciplines and specific projects" (Leonelli, 2012, p. 1). Yet even though facilitating exchange of materials is understood as a key purpose of biobanks, this is in most cases not entirely detached from the attachments at play in building a collection. One researcher brought this to a point by pointing out that the PI who controls the collection ultimately decides what can be shared or not.

As a centralized repository, the STN aimed to avoid these kinds of commitments. As one senior policy official mentioned, Singapore's main research funding agency A*STAR set up STN "[to] invite people to store" and in return for free storage "to make sure they shared samples with people who wanted to use them". Researchers interested in using materials stored in STN could apply with the network's steering committee, which would first consider the scientific merit of the proposed use and next whether sufficient material was still available to supply the requested amount. Access to STN samples, one researcher explained, followed STN rules, without requiring any recognition of the hospital the sample came from or any control for the initial contributor. Yet even though the person who had initially contributed the sample to STN could not influence who would be given access, they still had a lever. A policy official explained how all data remained with the PI and the PI would therefore have to be involved in order to make use of the materials possible. Judging by the references to limited use as a reason for closing STN and interview respondents' claims that they could not use the collection due to lack of data, clinicians and researchers collecting the data used this possibility to their advantage.[7]

However, when speaking of data sharing in interviews, researchers listed a much broader set of criteria for why (not) to make samples available to other researchers. When judging a request against the remaining amount of material available, researchers also have possible future need for materials in mind. One researcher therefore explained how the use of the material must be worthwhile and contribute to solving a "major question", or allow researchers to obtain measurements they would not otherwise be able to get. Requests are also subject to what one person described as "sample bargaining" or negotiations over the exact amount required and how much the repository is willing to give up. Moreover at one repository tied to a hospital, researchers from that hospital would be prioritized in getting access. External users would be required to collaborate with a staff member of the hospital. This criterion created a bit of a dilemma, since sample contributors would ideally be co-authors on any publications, even though for most scientific journals authorship requires more than supplying samples. This repository resolved this dilemma by insisting that the surgeon supplying the sample had also gathered the relevant data on its donor. The likelihood of getting to a publication too served as a criterion considered by the repository's access committee, thereby creating a more complicated puzzle for when and how to share materials than the STN did. One major difference seems to be that, by extending authorship, this repository gave contributors a way to benefit from sharing data.

These distinct approaches to when and how to share materials, as well as the persistent issue of financial sustainability indicate how imaginaries of (economically) productive collaboration around the STN did not fully align with researchers' views of a future for which the value of a collection should be carefully curated. This raises the question if and how different (kinds of) values were attributed to and enacted through STN's design and operations. To get a sense of an answer to this question, we will turn to the various tensions that ultimately contributed to the demise of STN next.

Practices of Purpose and the Closing of STN

Both in media commentary and in interviews, the reasons that were given for STN to be closed in 2011 often revolved around the issue of use (Chang, 2011; Chan, 2012). More specifically, a lack of use of the materials stored in what was by then known as Singapore Biobank (SBB) allegedly caused research funding agency A*STAR to reconsider its investment in the repository. At the time, SBB was not the only facility or institute established in the context of the Biomedical Sciences Initiative under such scrutiny. Across the biomedical research landscape, Singapore's government recalibrated its funding portfolio as the initiative entered its third 5-year phase, which had as its main aim to get (financial) returns on prior investments (Fischer, 2013; Nature, 2010). Considering these wider circumstances, it is not self-evident that "lack of use" was the only or even decisive reason for shutting SBB down (Aarden, 2017b). As one biobank manager explained to me, STN had a recovery rate (meaning the percentage of stored samples actually retrieved for research) of about 18%.[8] He did not further classify this number as either high or low, yet suggested that the order of magnitude of this rate is relatively common. This is why, in his view there is "consensus [that] government funding is required", while in Singapore "[the] government wants money back". This he described as "a Catch-22 situation".

Other interview respondents suggested that this Catch-22 had something to do with the broader "model" chosen for the Singapore Tissue Network and its costs relative to the overall biomedical research budget. One policy official linked his concern about low usage of available materials and the idea that nobody wanted to store tissue there with the observation that biobanking is "very expensive; it's not sustainable for Singapore". Another policy-maker agreed, arguing that once the collection started to grow with (especially) the inclusion of ever more blood samples from cohort studies, it started using up too large a portion of the country's overall research budget. At the same time, this person maintained that the collection was not particularly useful, since it remained too small to provide the individual number of samples required for genetic research on—especially—rare diseases. While claiming that biobanking is important, this person located STN's lack of success in the use of the wrong "model". Taking this idea a step further, a former STN staffer suggested that "they [presumably meaning the Singapore government] have not considered what kind of biobank they wanted. The objectives were not very clear". Rather than merely researchers being disinclined to use available materials, it thus seems that the usefulness of the biobank itself was put in question.

In the context of the STN as well as biobanking writ large, this notion of use is always related to circulation. Ideally, use of biobank materials involves other researchers than those who have collected the materials. Reflecting on the global circulation of data, Sabina Leonelli (2013) therefore observes how data (and tissue) expected to travel the globe are in that sense "bigger" than individual research projects. Repositories of tissue and data need to be suitable for facilitating (global) circulation by encompassing various possible research applications in how materials are processed and stored. As the case of the STN shows, this aim of circulation can stand in tension to issues of local interests and control. Various authors have therefore proposed to think of data exchange in terms of "data journeys" (Bates et al., 2016; Leonelli, 2016, 2020). Conceiving of how data moves in these terms allows analysts "to better situate data across interconnected sites of practice through time and space" (Bates et al., 2016, p. 2) and observe how "journeys are hardly ever unproblematic" (Leonelli, 2016, p. 40). Seeing the movement of data (and tissue) as a major objective of centralized storage in Singapore thus shifts attention from the question why materials were not used to what hindered these materials in (quite literally) moving from storage to use.

Earlier in this discussion we have seen how the "sticky issue" (to quote a former STN collaborator) of ownership formed an obstacle for contributing materials to the tissue network—let alone for using them. The same respondent argued that "the *quid pro quo* of giving and getting access" to tissue and data materials "took lots of negotiation" when STN was first established. As a solution to this problem STN developed a form of shared ownership or control of samples, expressed to what interview respondents referred to as the aforementioned "50–50 rule". This was an arrangement in which samples were stored in full at STN, but half of the sample would be exclusively available to the person who had contributed it, while the other half was available to any researcher putting a successful application to the STN steering committee.

However, researchers and clinicians contributing samples found another way to keep a degree of control over the use of samples, which was somewhat ironically facilitated by a design feature intended to engineer collaboration. When describing the set-up of STN, a former staff member described how the network also established a databank and a case report form for samples. This form included "minimal identifying data", which required a sample user to link to a principal investigator (PI) who had contributed the sample to make research "truly collaborative [...] and break down the barriers of competition in such a small country". Yet it is a truism of sorts among biobanking professionals that tissue is useless without detailed clinical data. Most therefore saw the absence of such data at STN itself as a deficit rather than an invitation. One researcher described the repository as "just like a middle man [having] some clinical information, but not the whole picture". Being somewhat more outspoken, a colleague described the availability of samples and "minimal" clinical data as "not very useful". Instead, he continued, deep clinical phenotyping would be required to use the materials in research. Without it, he classified STN as "a nice library with very little relevance".

While such design decisions and how they were perceived by potential users complicate "lack of use" as a cause of STN's closing, other responses to the question why this happened show how this issue was only the top of the proverbial iceberg. As noted above, budgetary constraints were one important issue. As one researcher argued somewhat facetiously, "it was a success for us, but not for Biobank, because every year they burned cash. Nothing happened to the samples, they were just stored there...". This person thereby again highlights a discrepancy between costs and use. In particular, he links a lack of use to the pharmaceutical industry's unwillingness to pay for using samples for, for example, product testing.[9] Additionally, a research administrator attributed financial concerns to the aforementioned recalibration of research funding for the third phase of the BMSI. At this point, he explained, A*STAR, which is responsible for funding basic research and had also financed STN, saw much of its budget shifted to the Ministry of Health, which primarily funds applied clinical and translational research. Presumably, this also meant that less funding was available for a centralized tissue repository.

Furthermore, this reference to shifting budgets makes clear how the fate of STN ties into broader characteristics of and changes in Singapore's research landscape. Against that background, a researcher responded to my question why the repository closed by describing its "failure" as "a symptom of a lot of things". Getting a bit more specific, he identified two major problems related to institutional aspects of research and health care in Singapore. On the one hand, he echoed concerns I had heard before about the government's top-down approach to biomedical research. As he framed it, the repository was designed without considering knowledge about biobanking "on the ground" and about implementation. On the other hand, he pointed to the organization of health care in Singapore into different hospital clusters that were expected to compete (Hasseltine, 2013). While he acknowledged the idea that this might contribute to decreasing health care costs, he also believed that it made expectations that the clusters would suddenly collaborate in research unlikely to succeed. The competition between clusters was indeed often cited as a challenge for research that the tissue network had been expected to help resolve. Both in the design of the repository and in the fragmentation of health care in Singapore this person therefore saw institutional constraints on STN's possible contributions to scientific collaboration.

Along with these institutional challenges, respondents described other difficulties they broadly described as "cultural". A subset of these issues related to the relation between clinicians and researchers. The location of STN on the Biopolis research campus, which, as several people pointed out to me, does not include hospitals, often seemed to be perceived as indicative of this issue. It was often described in terms of supposed "frictions" between clinicians and basic researchers and attributed particularly to distrust among clinicians regarding how researchers would use "their" samples. Additionally, some people felt that clinicians were jealous of the elevated status of (often foreign) laboratory scientists under the government's biomedical research investments. The significant role of established scientists recruited from abroad was supposedly another cause of friction and a reason why clinicians and local researchers remained sceptical towards the repository. One policy official, for example, described the Chinese-American director of STN's leadership style as a problem for making the repository work. Others turned this notion around and argued that much effort went into confronting resistance, addressing distrust of foreigners and the "heavily competitive, almost tribal" nature of research institutions in Singapore—although the person using this qualification described it as an "Asian" problem. While many of these accusations do not amount to much more than hearsay, they suggest that a complex range of issues—which at the very least turned out to be real in their effects—affected the Singapore Tissue Network. Some of these were woven into the repository design and the way it corresponded with specific purposes of tissue collection and storage. Others, however, seem to reflect broader conflicts and uncertainties within the rapidly expanding biomedical research landscape in Singapore.

In 2011, A*STAR concluded from these various issues that continued funding for a centralized tissue repository was no longer viable. As a policy official told me, this was a "rational decision" and involved returning samples and some equipment such as freezers to the country's research institutions. Yet, at the time I did research in Singapore—roughly 2 years after the fact—there was still lingering anger and confusion. Many researchers felt the decision had been sudden and unnecessary; others were still not entirely sure where all the samples they had collected ended up, or expressed concern about the long-term damage this decision might cause for biobanking in Singapore. By contrast, one senior policy official considered the decision not to have had a significant effect on the country's reputation as an emerging Asian hub for biomedical research. Indeed, about a decade later it seems that new efforts to create a national biobank have since been developed (Vimal et al., 2023). Nevertheless, the episode provides some insight into the different purposes and forms of value imagined for tissue repositories and how these may affect both the set-up of such research infrastructures and their "sustainability".

Conclusion: Contested Imaginaries and Value Making in a National Tissue Repository

In this chapter, I focused on how various *purposes* of infrastructures for population-based medical research were articulated in the design and operations of the Singapore Tissue Network (STN) as well as other tissue repositories in Singapore. Informed by different notions of imaginaries that project both broader sociopolitical ambitions onto science and technology and considering how such projects are reflected in scientific practice itself (McNeil et al., 2017) I traced a wide range of promises and expectations that informed biobanking in Singapore. The various imaginaries held by people and institutions involved in both research policies and practices commonly revolved around different kinds of value expected from biobanking. Following the lead of a research approach characterized as "valuography" (Dussauge et al., 2015b), I considered such values a product of various processes along the 'lifespan' of tissue samples, ranging from donor recruitment to scientific publication, but also as something designed or build into the (organizational) architecture of tissue repositories (Aarden, 2024). This approach enabled me to make the complex range of ideas, procedures and actions that informed various framings of the purposes of tissue repositories in Singapore visible. Ultimately, such a pragmatic approach allowed more fundamental insight into the differences between various repositories and provided a more complex answer to the question why STN closed than the oft-cited "lack of use".

The purposes of tissue repositories and the forms of value generation these are linked to can take many different forms. Purposes are often not explicitly articulated, but are embedded into how repositories are organized and operated. Both overall design of tissue repositories and the forms of "data (and tissue) labour" (Nadim, 2016) performed there reflect such an institution's purposes. These may also be in conflict, as the case of STN vividly shows. Both design and operations of the tissue network were geared towards specific purposes, formulated by the funding agency A*STAR in the context of Singapore's biomedical sciences initiative. STN was perceived as a support structure for this essentially economic initiative.

Based on the idea that collaborative research would be most likely to generate commercially promising outcomes, enabling collaboration was a key aim in setting up a centralized repository. STN's set-up therefore included a number of characteristics developed with this aim in mind. Most striking among them were free sample storage, the 50–50 sharing rule intended to increase contributions, and the absence of any significant clinical data. These characteristics have in common that they detach samples from specific contexts of collection and use. With hindsight, such detachment was problematic since for many researchers, their attachment to samples and data, as well as to the people they are expected to collaborate with, are important (Pinel & Svendsen, 2021). Researchers would also discuss recruitment of research participants, collection of samples and decision-making on whom to share with and how to acknowledge collaborators in ways that highlight the deeply situated nature of sample storage.

Against this background, the lack of influence on who would use samples and the absence of data came to be seen as 'mistakes' and as choosing the wrong model. However, such critiques cannot be seen separate from various other contextual factors, such as shifts in funding priorities, distrust within the research system and the fragmentation of Singapore's health care system, which all contributed to the end of STN to some degree.

Much social science critique of biomedical research in Singapore, then, is too sweeping in its characterization of its purposes and effects. Closer scrutiny of the multiple purposes of biobanking shows diversity and friction within the research landscape that cannot easily be reduced to singular factors (e.g., the dominance of foreign scientists). The tensions around centralized tissue storage in Singapore that emerged over time reflect both issues that are typical of biobanking in other places as well as specific issues related to the complex architecture of biomedical research in Singapore. The question of long term (financial) sustainability of individual biobanks, for example, is widely discussed (Watson et al., 2014; Doucet et al., 2017). Similarly, struggles over ownership of samples and data as well as researchers' reluctance to share materials have been analysed in various studies of the social dynamics of biobanking elsewhere (Tupasela, 2017a, 2021; Sandor, 2009). Even the closing of biobanks due to the unclear status of samples and disappointed expectations about collections' purposes and value are not unique to Singapore (Stephens & Dimond, 2015a, b).

The virtually global coverage of some of the biobanking issues affecting STN also suggests that references to "Asian culture" may be overblown. Nevertheless, there are some locally specific factors that contributed to the difficulties for STN. Some of these may be framed as yet another line of conflict between various purposes; not just around the question how attached clinicians and researchers can and should be to their materials, but also around the complex architecture of a repository not directly tied into, but largely dependent on, a health care system geared towards competition. Here, a sense of distrust among clinicians towards the now suddenly more prominent researchers that some respondents mentioned intersects with the respectively collaborative and competitive purposes designed into medical science and medical care. If a design flaw is the key to the closing of STN, it is possibly not just a flaw in usefulness, but also in the misalignment of research and health care.

These observations do not imply that researchers in Singapore stand opposed to policy-makers, or 'the lab' is pitted against 'the clinic'. Most researchers I interviewed acknowledged and accepted that technical innovation and economic growth are the main motivations for their research being funded to begin with. Not to mention that the line is blurry and many researchers at some point take on a policy-making or administrative role. Similarly, research and health care are not completely separate categories. Moreover, practices of research participant recruitment and sample collection intersect with care work—even for cohort studies, where participants are not already enrolled in a health care setting. Such care work serves the purpose of growing the pool of participants and donors, but is in turn entangled with particular social relations regarding, for instance, the treatment of the elderly in Singapore.

The purposes of medical research in Singapore took on a number of different forms, and gave rise to a diverse set of "valuation" practices (Dussauge et al., 2015a). These practices do not follow by necessity from the logic of value making in the life sciences—which are furthermore not clear cut or uniform to begin with (Birch & Tyfield, 2013; Chiapetta & Birch, 2018). Rather, the pursuit of value in tissue and data storage in Singapore is shaped by sociotechnical imaginaries (Jasanoff & Kim, 2009, 2015) of national identity and cohesion built through state-led economic development (Lee, 2007; Trocki, 2009). This observation aligns with the idea that expectations and promises are constitutive of the life sciences and biomedical research at the beginning of the twenty-first century (Martin, 2018). But it also shows how the realization of such promises and imaginaries is heavily contested in practice and confronted with the technoscientific imaginaries (Marcus, 1995) that inform scientific practice. In the multiple purposes of medical research collections, we find the materiality of research practices and science governance tied together in ways that may cause an infrastructure to be established as well as deconstructed. How different infrastructures may also exist at the same time and thereby shape distinct approaches to a population will be the topic of the next chapter.

Notes

1. Other examples included questioning about what had happened (in terms of publications) with the roughly 40 requests for samples since 2009, or the insistence that two surgeons who were the main sources of lymphoma samples should be included as authors on any publications based on work with these samples. We will return to the specific dynamics of biomedical research that inform these moments later in the chapter.
2. The name change was more than just cosmetic, as it reflected a shift from a repository primarily containing 'solid' tissue samples to one that consisted primarily of 'liquid' blood samples. This shift had far-reaching consequences for the repository that played a significant role in its termination. While the rebranding lasted for a relatively short time, I have not been able to pinpoint when this change occurred, exactly.
3. Some would go even further back arguing that, even as a British colony "Singapore was established for economic reasons" (Trocki, 2009, p. 6; see also Lee, 2007).
4. It is an open question whether the success of such policies—at least in terms of sustained long-term economic growth—reflect the idea that the nation of Singapore "works" or are merely the logical outcome of the country's profitable geographical location and other resources. See (Neher, 1999) and (Lingle & Wickman, 1999) for both sides of this debate.
5. Although Edwin Lee (2008) presents a counterargument by describing Singapore as an "unexpected nation" that unintentionally emerged from this continuous process of economic development and explicitly not as the expression of any "imagined community" (to use Anderson's (2006) concept).
6. And, as various respondents added, was prime real estate that was possibly too expensive for storing tissue.
7. As a matter of speaking. It is a different debate to what extent not sharing data is advantageous and to whom.
8. For more on cost recovery in biobanking, see (Clément et al., 2014).
9. It is, however, unclear how realistic a source of financing this was. Another person told me how sample uses was limited to basic research as part of efforts to address scepticism among clinicians to contribute samples to the repository.

4

Making Population in Accounting for Mortality in the Million Death Study

Around the time the calendar turned from 2013 to 2014, I visited three cities in India to interview (mostly) researchers and government officials about the Million Death Study (MDS), an effort to generate cause-specific mortality statistics for India (Jha, 2014; Jha et al., 2006). The study was set up as a solution for the alleged deficiencies in civil registration of causes of death in the Indian population. As one interview respondent summarized the problem at one point, officially certified causes of death in India were "urban-based, hospital-based, and often not the right cause of death". This suggests both that civil registration is not reliable and that in the many cases of people dying at home in rural areas, deaths are not registered at all. To confront these issues, the MDS makes use of a method called verbal autopsy (VA), using household interviews conducted in the context of an existing infrastructure for monitoring population dynamics, the Sample Registration System (SRS). Keeping to a brief summary for now, whenever a dead is reported in the SRS sample, the government enumerator collecting this data would be required to ask a set of questions geared towards gathering descriptions of symptoms preceding this person's death. On the basis of such symptomatic data, physicians subsequently determine individual cause of death. All individual causes then get aggregated to generate statistics on the

E. Aarden, *Producing Citizenship in Medical Research Collections*, Health, Technology and Society, https://doi.org/10.1007/978-981-95-1707-7_4

cause-specific distribution of mortality in the Indian population as a whole. Both the verbal autopsy method and its result are consequently considered to enable health policy improvements and to be able to serve as a model for the global South.

As several of my respondents explained to me how the study worked, what purposes it served and what its main challenges were, one characterization in particular stood out to me. A software developer for the study assured me it was "all about big data and how it can provide evidence of the health problems in developing countries". This seemed a peculiar description of the MDS to me. I had not considered any similarity between this study, which interview respondents regularly described in terms of its low costs and simple approach, and the rapid processing of large amounts of digital data. Nevertheless, I propose to take this description seriously as an analytical entry point and to explore how the 'datafication' (Mejias & Couldry, 2019) of mortality in this study might be understood. As I will discuss below, issues such as data quality and processing play an important role. The study also seems to be at least in part informed by ideas akin to the view that large amounts of data facilitate knowledge production independent of formulating theories and testing hypotheses (Kitchin, 2014a). This particular understanding of and approach to data in the study of population mortality further serves to understand the MDS as an infrastructure for the purpose of *population-based* medical research. In particular, it foregrounds how population gets captured in the form of data. More specifically, I am interested here in the particular ways a presumed (national) population gets broken down into a research object and a set of data points allowing diagnostics before getting pieced back together into a population with a specific profile of (the distribution of) mortality.

Statistics and quantification in the context of (global) public health have long been subjects of social science analysis. Brown et al. (2012), for example, argue that technologies of knowledge production and their intersections with mechanisms of government are key to contemporary global health. The particular epistemic and organizational configuration of the MDS may be considered a fairly straightforward example of the emerging field of global health (see, e.g., Aarden, 2021; Birbeck et al., 2013). It enacts an epistemic approach to health and disease that David Reubi (2018) has aptly described as "epidemiological reason", in which an emphasis on a defined population, rigorous epidemiological data and the aim to save as many lives as possible are key. However, in this chapter I wish to further explore the entanglements between definitions of a population and the generation of epidemiological statistics by engaging with critical perspectives on the making of data and classifications (boyd & Crawford, 2012; Iliadis & Russo, 2016). A central tenet of my argument is that population and health get mediated through the making and processing of data. I will trace this mediating role of data through the details of knowledge production in the MDS below.

In this chapter, I trace how particular versions of India and of the health of India's population are produced through the datafication of mortality. To trace processes of data production, circulation and interpretation, I will first turn to the question how a population is made through particular sampling and data collection methods. I draw on the work of Michel Foucault and historians of statistics here to reconstruct how India's population is constructed as a knowledge object in the making of the SRS sample. Next, I will shift my attention from the SRS in general to the Million Death Study as such to investigate the procedures and criteria through which symptomatic data points are extracted from this population sample. I link this analysis to a wider discussion of different meanings of and promises and expectations attached to data. Next, I turn to the use and classification of symptomatic datapoints to diagnose individual causes of death, focusing on how the particular aims of the study shape these classifications. I further explore how the resulting, individual causes of death are re-aggregated into a population that thereby becomes an object of governance. I will highlight how this involves particular interpretations of what matters about the previously produced diagnoses and what not. In conclusion, I will discuss how the construction of a population involves the construction of particular notions of what matters about health and disease as expressed through data.

Making a Population Through Data

The MDS started around the turn of the Millennium as an effort to generate representative and reliable cause of death statistics for the Indian population. Such statistics are considered vital for formulating adequate public health policies (see, e.g., Deaton, 2013). As one of the study initiators told me in an interview, when he and a colleague started thinking about the study, "what we found in vital registration is that at the national level, at state levels, these estimates [of causes of death] were not possible". Several other initiatives to collect causal mortality statistics had been in place, different researchers told me, including cause of death reporting by relatives (without professional medical certification) and the medical certification of causes of death, which covered about 75% of all hospital deaths. Yet these supposedly form only a minority of deaths—as yet another person told me, most people in India, and in low and middle income countries in general, die at home, in rural areas, without any medical attention. The absence of cause of death data is thus (in part) framed as a shortcoming of India's medical system. It is therefore not insignificant that the study was initiated by a medical researcher and a demographer, reflecting how demographic and medical research infrastructures would tie together in the study. Furthermore, there is an emphasis in the study on data that is considered 'routine', describing what people die from on average. The collection of such data, then, is said to require "ruthless discipline in objectivity, measurement and in priority setting" (World Health Organization, 2010).

The study's focus on undiagnosed deaths and hypotheses about an ongoing epidemiological transition and "residual" burden of infectious diseases in particular suggest a focus on the lower end of India's socioeconomic curve. This is not to deny that there is widespread—if often marginalized (Prasad, 2014b)—investment in research on the frontiers of biomedicine and biotechnology in India, which has received considerable attention in the social sciences (see, e.g., Sunder Rajan, 2012, 2017). Yet, India remains an important site of global health intervention and experimentation as well, and is sometimes—including in the MDS—seen as an exemplar for lower income countries elsewhere. This 'global health' focus (Brown et al., 2006; Birn, 2009; McGoey et al., 2011) is also reflected in the organization and funding of the study. Apart from the Office of the Registrar General of India (RGI), which manages the SRS, it involves institutions both in India and elsewhere. This includes research institutions—the study is coordinated by the Centre for Global Health Research at the University of Toronto in Canada, but also involves various Indian research institutions—as well as national research funding agencies in India, Canada, the United States and the Gates Foundation.

Part of the interest of this wide variety of institutions in the study originates from its efforts at epidemiological innovation, not least in the form of increasingly rigorous, standardized and decontextualized interventions and metrics (Adams, 2013, 2016). Efforts to assure the aforementioned "rigorous discipline" in the MDS rely on two innovations in comparison to the registration of deaths in the health system, which is widely characterized as deeply deficient in India (Global Health Watch, 2011; Drèze & Sen, 2013; Chowdhury, 2015). One innovation concerned the use of symptomatic data gathered through the so-called verbal autopsy method. According to its description in the study manual, this method "involves a household assessment of the causes of death, which is an investigation of train of events and circumstances at the onset and during the course of illness leading to death, through an interview of relatives or associates of the deceased" (SRS Collaborators of the RGI-CGHR, 2011, p. 2). The study thereby avoids reliance on either hospital diagnoses or causes of death assigned by relatives and instead seeks to piece together causes of death from the "data points" (Armstrong, 2019) describing symptoms and collected in household interviews. A second innovation serves to avoid problems of representativeness by using a population sample independent of hospitals and other medical institutions, called the Sample Registration System (SRS).

The SRS, described as "the largest demographic survey in the world" (Office of the Registrar General of India, 2013), is operated by the Office of the Registrar General of India (ORGI), which also runs the full decennial census. According to one interview respondent, the SRS was developed in the 1960s on the basis of the observation that the population had grown much more than expected during the decade-long interval of the full population census. This person claimed that such unexpected growth illustrated the need for more fine-grained annual assessment of population dynamics. These are therefore traced in a representative sample of the full population, which is revised every 10 years on the basis of the full census. The SRS sample includes so-called enumeration blocks selected to be representative of rural areas, villages, towns and larger cities. The total sample consists of a little less than 1% of India's population, which, at the time of my interviews, still included about 8 million people. At the time, the full sample included 8861 units consisting of 1000–1500 people. The SRS uses a so-called double enumeration procedure. This means that all relevant changes in a sample unit's population—births, deaths and migration—are first recorded by a local enumerator. This is often a school teacher or nurse who is familiar with the area. In addition to such continuous enumeration, a government official conducts retrospective enumeration, collecting the same information from household visits once every 6 months. Data collection for the Million Death Study is attached to this retrospective enumeration.

SRS units are defined at the state level and allow statistically significant extrapolations at the national and state level, as well as between urban and rural areas—but not at a smaller scale. In an interview at the demographic office in one of the Indian states, a demographer used the map of a small village to explain how SRS units were defined—something he was tasked with at the time (in early 2014), as the new sample based on the 2011 census needed to be implemented soon. He explained how new units should consist of less than 2000 inhabitants, which meant that towns like the one on the map he showed needed to be divided into smaller units. Defining these units, he explained, required quite a bit of work. They would be based on housing blocks as well as local landmarks to help enumerators identify the boundaries of a unit. In addition, an inventory of houses in the blocks would be needed to make sure any changes (like the demolition of a house) would not be mischaracterized as changes in population. Finally, enumerators needed to make sure to count only people belonging to households that are part of the sample (and not, e.g., visitors). For this purpose, households were defined as people taking food from a common kitchen and spending a certain amount of time in the house. This way, the SRS creates a particular definition of who belongs to the population, which gets standardized to be 'legible' (Scott, 1999) over time.

In a similar vein, the overall size of the sample uses the census as a framework, but is based on criteria for identifying "events of interest". Put simply, in order to make statistically tenable claims about certain events, enough of these events need to occur in the sample to be able to extrapolate to the full population. The least common of the events of interest therefore shapes the required sample size. For the SRS, the main event of interest had long been maternal mortality, one person explained to me. But because this occurred less and less frequently, it was no longer feasible to operate a sample on this basis. The least common event shaping the sample had therefore been changed to infant mortality, with maternal mortality estimates now being made once every 3 years. The same logic also caused one researcher to admit to having some reservations about the use of the SRS in the MDS. He explained how the parameters for defining sampling units do not include disease incidence, causing some regionally prevalent diseases to be either overlooked or overrepresented. Yet, he added not to consider this a big issue, since "still it is better than having nothing at all". As we will see below, both the issue of the sample's shortcomings and the notion that it is better than nothing resonate throughout the study.

As a vast body of historical and sociological research has shown, the census—and by extension an infrastructure such as the SRS—has long served to both make populations and make them visible in specific ways. Especially pertinent to the case presented here, Bernard Cohn (1987, 1996) has observed how the census in colonial British India served as both a tool of knowledge and of power, forming an effort by the British to understand and control India by rendering it in numerical form. This perspective resonates with the rather more sweeping claims Foucault has made with regard to the historical emergence of population as an object of government. Foucault, too, diagnoses the mutual configuration of population as an object of knowledge and government, pointing to statistics and normal distributions as ways of defining objects of government (Foucault, 2007, 2013; Lemke, 2007). Recent work building on Foucault's notions of biopower and biopolitics in the context of (global) public health has argued that "truth discourses" and means of intervention in population have shifted from the burdens of disease and death to assessments of quality of life (Wahlberg & Rose, 2015; Villadsen & Wahlberg, 2015; Rabinow & Rose, 2006), although the case of the Million Death Study suggests that such a perspective may overestimate these shifts beyond the global North (Clarke et al., 2010). Moreover, in studying the historical emergence of the Canadian census, Bryan Curtis has questioned Foucault's conceptualization of population. Rather than understanding population as an object of knowledge and intervention, he proposes to see it as "a way of organizing social observations" (Curtis, 2002, p. 24). This perspective suggests that population is itself a product of knowledge production processes and is made up in conjunction with the formation of the state. Foreshadowing our later discussion of population rendered as data, Curtis (2002, p. 33) maintains that the census is *made* rather than taken.

Other analysts of what I would describe as the production of population have made similar observations, scrutinizing both what population refers to and the procedures, devices and practices through which it gets made. Michelle Murphy (2017, p. 7) has described population as a "material-semiotic-affective infrastructural" phenomenon, summarizing the various ways population gets constructed and can be present in the world, based on techniques, discourses, representations, imaginations, etc., while also forming a basis for other forms of knowledge and intervention. Population can thus be understood as something that "is rarely defined [...] except in abstract statistical terms" (Krieger, 2012, p. 635) and has thus "come to acquire a technical meaning" (Krieger, 2012, p. 639). At the same time, population is an object "of imagination, knowledge and governing" (Grommé & Ruppert, 2019, p. 255) and based on epistemic assumptions about population logics (Moreira, 2019), constructed and knowable through various calculative devices. To understand how population is made through data, I therefore trace both the material and imaginative forms of its construction in the MDS.

The making of population by means of particular routines and devices always revolves around the making of similarity and difference. The construction of population involves "identifying common characteristics that bring different individuals into sameness [while] in the process delinking parts of individuals from other parts of themselves and from their social context(s)" (Biruk, 2022, p. 313). Both the integrative (making sameness) and disintegrative (delinking) dimensions of population are shaped through the particular techniques and devices of making population. Cal Biruk, for example, has shown the work that is required on the ground to make data for an epidemiological research project (Biruk, 2012). While the making of a (quantified) population always simultaneously involves the making of the state, a focus on practices and techniques of quantifying a population (i.e., statistics) shows how "the state" always remains an unfinished project that can take on different shapes through the formation of different governing relations (Callon & Latour, 1981; Das & Poole, 2004). This becomes particularly visible when considering the SRS and MDS in India. Not only is the state's role in counting the population translated into counting a sample to get a better grasp of short term population dynamics (in the SRS), the state's responsibility for population health is enacted as a demographic rather than medical issue by virtue of the MDS' data collection method. This demographic reading of population health in turn requires turning medical conditions into "data points" (Armstrong, 2019) suitable for further processing and quantification.

Delving into the mechanisms that turn the Indian population into a cumulative set of causes of death via the SRS shows how—after Murphy—population is made in material-semiotic and affective form. A starting point for thinking through the framing of population health in the MDS might be to ask the question why the focus is on causes of death. This is not only due to—to quote one study researcher—"how important understanding causes of death is to improving health of the living". It is also because death is a good entry point for making population health visible, especially since data collection through verbal autopsy starts with relatives and government enumerators without medical training. One researcher explains how:

> symptoms are very pronounced and defined at time of death. So the only thing is, if you are able to capture symptoms and events before the death, then the physician would be able to describe cause of death.

Verbal autopsy thus starts with attaching a particular meaning to population health, which is captured in terms of causes of death and made visible through specific techniques. These include material artefacts such as a data collection form and—further down the line—software platforms for data analysis. But it also includes a particular data collection technique that requires extensive training of government enumerators as well as standardized control and resampling mechanisms.

The description of populations through the quantitative technique of statistics produces or enacts the population in particular ways, forming "a way of drawing things together and holding them apart" (Cool, 2022, p. 334). Devices for making particular similarities and differences visible play a key role in different enactments of populations, and "different devices enact different populations as objects of concern and intervention" (Ruppert, 2011, p. 219). A key device for verbal autopsy data collection, for example, is the form the enumerator uses. There are four (slightly) different forms (called 10A through D) for neonatal, child, adult and maternal deaths, respectively. In addition to some basic administrative data (e.g., SRS unit number, date of interview, names of both the respondent and the deceased), the form includes a number of questions for gathering demographic and medical data. These include items such as age, marital status and education level, medical history and behaviour such as alcohol and tobacco consumption. The form also features half a page for writing a 'narrative'. This narrative is the main source of diagnostic data, with answers to most of the other questions used for confirmation. Although there is interest in the MDS in supplying all enumerators with tablets for direct data entry, at the time of my fieldwork the study still used paper forms that needed to be scanned and uploaded to a government server. They thus entered a broader set of administrative, sociotechnical relations which—so we will see—form as significant a part of the study's data practices as enumerators' data entry in the field (cf. Ruppert & Scheel, 2021).

Accurate data entry in the field is seen as a critical condition for the study to work. The study has therefore spent quite some resources on instructing enumerators on how to gather and control data. One example thereof is a training video that breaks the task of the enumerator down into five steps, drawing a comparison with the steps Indian cricket legend Sachin Tendulkar supposedly took for any batting turn.[1] These steps include, first, for the enumerator to listen to the respondent. To then get useful data from listening, the second step involves asking about so-called positive symptoms (the ones a person had before dying) and, in a third step, to further "probe the symptoms" and ask for specific details about, for instance, duration and sequence. To support the enumerators, the study has developed a list of 12 so-called cardinal symptoms that ought to be considered—including things like fever, vomiting, jaundice, etc. In a fourth step, the enumerator should make sure to exclude symptoms the deceased did not have (called negative symptoms) by asking about them specifically. The final step is then to "put it all together" into a narrative that can be entered on the form, confirming the sequence of events once more with the VA-respondent. By following these steps, enumerators are thus expected to generate symptomatic data that, in a next step, facilitates diagnosis of a person's cause of death. Before being used for diagnosis, all forms undergo automated quality control. The quality of data collection is further also controlled via re-sampling of 5% of all deaths, for which the verbal autopsy interview is repeated.

These steps reflect how researchers in the MDS imagine the population to become a knowledge object, particularly relative to the perceived insufficiencies of medical registration. The circumstance that causes of death are not adequately (or representatively) captured within the health care system is considered to be a major obstacle in producing population-wide mortality statistics. Attaching the MDS to the SRS is a first step towards solving this problem. With the aid of verbal autopsy, this demographic sample can also be a medical sample, yet to avoid biases and preliminary conclusions, the demographic sample is enacted primarily as an object of medical knowledge—indeed a collection of data points rather than a collection of subjects with medical conditions. This means that, as one researcher explained, "the staff is consciously not medically trained, since they are comparable to medical students who are taught to listen and record without drawing conclusions". Their task is to "capture the information, getting accurate information without a bias towards a particular diagnosis". Enumerators thereby serve as a kind of symptomatic "sensors" for the study (Aarden, 2021).

At the same time, researchers place significant emphasis on the particular value of collecting data through household interviews in the context of the SRS. One person described as "[t]he kernel of everything" the "respectful conversation between two adults, in which they ask what happened". Someone else emphasized how "it can't be done like a research methodology. It has to be integrated in the system", due to the number of enumerators required for data collection. Not only the symptomatic data points as such, but also how these can be collected form a critical part of how a population can be made.

After a few years piloting the method, data collection and 'coding' of symptomatic narratives started in earnest in 2001. I was told that about 50,000 forms are filled out each year, out of which 40 to 45,000 can be coded—the rest is either incomplete or not of sufficient quality. From the forms that qualify, narratives of the circumstances surrounding death become rendered as data for diagnosing cause of death. Before turning to the question how symptoms become diagnoses, I therefore want to consider the question what 'data' comes to mean in this context. As Rob Kitchin has suggested in his comprehensive discussion of the meaning(s) of data, they "are commonly understood to be the raw material produced by abstracting the world into categories, measures and other representational forms [...] that constitute the building blocks from which information and knowledge are created" (Kitchin, 2014b, p. 1). In the specific context of science, data may thus be "any product of research activities [...] that is collected stored, and disseminated *in order to be used as evidence for knowledge claims*" (Leonelli, 2016, p. 77). Both this definition and many further studies of (scientific) data practices have suggested that data is never 'raw' but always shaped by contexts of production, processing and use. Data are relational, enacting specific realities and exercising power (Kitchin, 2014b; Iliadis & Russo, 2016; Ruppert et al., 2017; Parry & Greenhough, 2018). Perhaps most importantly, data are also selective, attaching priority to certain (i.e., symptomatic) ways of describing death in the narratives.

Data are not only shaped by specific contexts, but can also be multiple and mean, be and do different things at the same time. Klaus Hoeyer (2023, p. 215) therefore proposes to think through data in terms of paradoxes, particularly with regard to how "investments in data do not always deliver, and sometimes what they do deliver is curiously different from what the promises suggested". Since, as Hoeyer suggests, "[p]romises lie at the heart of contemporary data politics" (Hoeyer, 2023, p. 31), it is worthwhile to consider data in the Million Death Study in terms of promise. How the Indian population is enacted through medical data that takes on different shapes and forms throughout the Million Death Study promises to supply more reliable cause of death statistics. Yet data also are and do other things in the context of the study. In that regard, I consider it useful to also consider the mobility of data—what some analysts have characterized as "data journeys" (Bates et al., 2016; Leonelli,

2016, 2020). This notion seeks to emphasize "the socio-material *life of data* as they travel between and through different sites of data practice" (Bates et al., 2016, p. 3). Even though this usually involves travel between different studies and institutions, raising questions on how to use data created for a different purpose, I suggest that thinking of data (enacting population) at different sites *within* the MDS can be fruitful, too. In particular, I suggest that thinking of data multiplicity and paradoxes as they travel can make visible how data's multiplicity frames population health in particular ways, leaving other options unexplored.

Classifying Narratives Towards Diagnosis

The generation of symptomatic narratives about any deaths occurring within an established population sample in India forms the first step in circumventing the deficiencies of the health system and civil registration and towards producing reliable and representative causal mortality statistics. The next step is to be able to determine what caused each individual death from data that was deliberately collected by people without medical training. To this end the MDS includes an intricate procedure for 'coding' the narratives that involves both a number of specified steps and two software platforms. Regarding the latter, the forms sent to the Office of the Registrar General of India (RGI), which operates the SRS, are first uploaded to a quality assessment platform. Here, entries on the form are controlled for whether the data is clean, consistent and complete and whether the language used matches the language code entered on the form (the MDS enables the use of eighteen recognized Indian languages).

Forms that are approved are then moved to the Central Medical Evaluation (CME) platform. This platform contains both a part where physicians invited to code the form can actually access it, as well as a part that coordinates the distribution of "records" (completed forms) on the basis of a language match and availability (since any physician can only have ten "open" records at the same time). In total, the study works with a panel of (at the time) around 300 physicians that code records for a small financial compensation per record—which at the time was eighteen rupees, or about the equivalent of one US dollar.

The coding process consists of a maximum of three steps. In a first step, two physicians code independently—which means that each of them attaches a diagnosis based on the International Classification of Diseases (ICD-10) to a death. For quality control purposes, physicians are also asked to assess the quality of the record and their degree of certainty about their own diagnosis. If the two physicians agree, this is the final step and the agreed-upon diagnosis is registered as the cause of death. If not, a second step called reconciliation follows. Here, the physicians receive each other's diagnosis and are asked to independently reconsider. In response, they may stick to their decision, accept the alternative proposed by their colleague, or decide on something different altogether. If this still does not result in a shared diagnosis, a third step called adjudication follows. In this step, a third, senior physician receives the two diagnoses and is asked to decide on a final diagnosis. This person can decide for one of the two given diagnoses or propose a different one on the basis of the available symptomatic information.

Physicians on the panel are expected to distil potentially relevant symptomatic information from the narratives they receive. One interview respondent, for example, showed me a narrative on his laptop screen and pointed to terms such as "swelling of the legs" as an example of key diagnostic data. In addition, physicians receive various instructions on how to go about coding. A key element here is that the production of representative statistics requires a focus on the most *common* causes of death. In the study manual for physicians, members of the panel are thus encouraged to "use common sense and best clinical judgement" to determine a cause of death on the basis of the (non-clinical) symptomatic data available (SRS Collaborators of the RGI-CGHR, 2011, p. 30).

To arrive at what is characterized as a "one death-one cause situation" (SRS Collaborators of the RGI-CGHR, 2011, p. 9), physicians are instructed to distinguish between the particular disease or *condition* initiating the "train of events" leading to death and what is called the *terminal event* and *risk factors* contributing to a condition. To clarify the difference, the study manual (SRS Collaborators of the RGI-CGHR, 2011, p. 11) describes as one of several examples the case of an elderly woman who slipped and fell, was bed-ridden with a broken leg, developed pneumonia and died. In this case, the correct ICD-10 code to register would be

W01—fall on the same level from slipping, tripping and stumbling—with pneumonia presumably only forming the terminal event. In an interview, one former study researcher now working for a government agency emphasized the imperfections of this approach by contrasting verbal autopsy's "aim to find causes of death" with diagnosis based on biological markers that would make it possible to "find out what is really happening". Along these lines, the Million Death Study is commonly described as an estimate, rather than any definitive determination of causes of death.

Estimates on a population level are based on aggregate individual diagnoses. To generate the latter, the study does not only follow a three-step diagnostic procedure or provide a set of instructions to its panel of coding physicians. These physicians are also supported by the aforementioned Central Medical Evaluation (CME) software platform. This platform supplies coding physicians with suggestions for a diagnosis on the basis of keywords physicians identify in a narrative. It may also suggest that a physician's chosen diagnosis is unlikely to be correct or even block certain diagnoses (for which one researcher mentioned a diagnosis of prostate cancer in female deaths as an example). These suggestions, so one researcher explained, mean that "the physician is being guided to assign an accurate diagnosis". Explaining this function, a software developer referred to the guidance for physicians as "metadata", which this person described as "this intellectual know-how we have built up over the years [from coding by physicians]", which is "incorporated into our system". Past diagnoses based on a particular set of symptoms are thus used to streamline and/or improve diagnosis in the present. The study thus contains a set of rules, routines and techniques aimed at arriving at accurate diagnoses, which simultaneously increasingly decontextualize symptoms from individual persons who have died.

The particular steps and concerns that inform the 'coding' of verbal autopsy data show diagnosis to be a socially shaped process (Jutel, 2011). Diagnosis is a process of classification that has the aim to find both similarities and differences between different instances of disease. It is central in attributing a specific status to medical conditions and detaching them from the individual sufferer—especially in situations such as the Million Death Study aimed at producing aggregate statistics of diseases and mortality. "Diagnosis", historian of medicine Charles Rosenberg (2002, p. 240) therefore writes, "is central to the definition and management of the social phenomenon that we call disease". What is worth highlighting in this description is, first, that diagnosis is not only a question of identification, but also of management and thus intervention, and, second, how disease is described as a social phenomenon. This suggests that both the definition of health conditions, but also their causes and possible responses cannot be seen separate from particular social affordances and limitations in making disease into a matter of (collective) concern.

A key dimension of the social processes that frame disease in the context of the MDS is the question which differences come to matter—or not—in relation to the verbal rather than biomedical description of symptoms. Which differences matter is essentially a question of classification. As Geoffrey Bowker and Susan Leigh Star (1999) have observed in their classic study of classification *Sorting Things Out*, classification systems and their categories are shaped by historical and social processes and decisions, but become naturalized over time, imbued with the assumption that classifications describe things—and their similarities, differences, and relations—as they are. Through their strategy of inversion, however, they read existing categories backwards to reconstruct how the taken for granted has come into being.

To do so, Bowker and Star take the International Classification of Diseases (ICD-10), which also structures the description of causes of death in the MDS, as one of their case studies. In their description, this classification is a pragmatic system that was created to serve particular purposes of identification and organization of diseases. ICD codes and their affiliated descriptions of disease thereby tell particular stories of what was considered medically relevant—not only in a scientific sense, but also for the purpose of identifying and addressing key issues for public health governance. Thus, Bowker and Star (1999, p. 118) write, "[b]uilding the ICD involved building the state as much as developing medical knowledge". Indeed, this is not only a way to make sense of the historical development of the ICD. I have already observed how the MDS, which involves the allocation of ICD codes on the basis of limited, non-clinical symptomatic data, is (also) an effort of (re-)building the Indian state in light of a deficient medical system. In this context, so a report on early MDS findings maintains (Office of the Registrar General of India, 2009), this alternative way of gathering data is essential for informing state efforts such as the planning of health programmes and evaluation of interventions.

In light of the diagnostic limitations of VA and the study's aims to inform health policy-making, its diagnostic classifications diverge slightly from the level of detail provided by the ICD. For individual diagnoses, study initiators have considered which diagnostic codes in the ICD may be considered 'equivalent' in light of the relatively coarse diagnostic distinctions verbal autopsy data permits as well as of the (lack of) distinction in what would be accurate health policy responses. Thus, one senior researcher explained the principle of these so-called "equivalent codes" to me on the basis of the diagnostic differentiation of diarrhoea. As he explained,

> A00 to A09 are the ICDs for diarrhoea. Different kinds of diarrhoea. But VA is not like in the clinic, where you diagnose things, so we say it is diarrhoea. So, if they [coding physicians] agree it is A00 to A09, in this range, we accept it [as the same diagnosis].

These equivalent codes have been programmed into the software. In most cases, the particular form of diarrhoea does not matter. Yet the database does retain the two different codes assigned by different physicians and reconsiders these at a later stage in the analysis. The same researcher explained to me how, at that stage, a different algorithm would apply a set of "trumping rules" to decide between the two codes. One of them is then used for further statistical analysis and the grouping of diagnoses into aggregate mortality statistics—all while keeping the limitations of verbal autopsy data in mind.

Although getting from symptomatic data to an accurate diagnosis required medical expertise and judgement, the notion of equivalence suggests that diagnoses remain somewhat uncertain. At the time of my interviews, the ability to diagnose was still a predominantly human skillset. This did happen with technological support, which was in turn interpreted as the beginning of a process in which human physicians could eventually be replaced. Nevertheless, while several diagnostic algorithms were tried on the data, "the current conclusion is [that] none of these are—not yet—well enough developed to replace the physician" as a software developer told me (see also Desai et al., 2014; Leitao et al., 2014). For some of the medical researchers involved, this was because "the computer lacks the physician's knowledge, it will not go into the fever's history or correlate with other symptoms". Yet others believed that machine learning, "which is not just that the machine is coding, but the machine itself is getting smarter as it codes" would take over at some point.

This idea resonates with a rhetoric of big data, albeit with comparatively minor volume. Yet key researchers' imagination of moving the human "out of the loop" (to invert a common phrase from the ethics of machine learning) extended beyond diagnosis. Since enumeration and coding are the most expensive parts of the study, there was quite some effort spent on how to replace people with machines. Whereas several studies of algorithms used in public services have shown the risks of bias and errant outcomes when presuming that machines can do a better, more accurate and more efficient job than human beings (O'Neil, 2016; Eubanks, 2017), an additional risk for public health in India seems to be that the complex problem of the country's burden of disease can be reduced to statistics and technicalities. To some degree, this risk is built into the study's framing of health as a statistical-scientific rather than political problem. This becomes apparent when we consider how population mortality statistics are distilled from aggregate individual diagnoses and how these are positioned to inform health programmes and policy.

From Diagnoses to Population Health Policy

The infrastructure of gathering cause of death data that circumvents medical diagnosis and civil registration in the MDS has ultimately been established to get better insight into the prevalence and distribution of cause-specific mortality in India. Knowing the most common causes of death in a population is widely seen as a key measure for improving public health overall (Jha, 2012; Deaton, 2013). We have thus far seen how both a *population* of interest is formed through the specific sampling and enumeration strategies of the Sample Registration System (SRS) and how *individual causes of death* are constructed through the collection of symptomatic data with the verbal autopsy method and diagnostic procedures applied by a panel of physicians. Yet the combination of a sample consisting of not quite 1% of India's population and the flexibility in interpreting symptoms (e.g., reflected in the use of equivalent ICD-codes) raises the question if and how the data produced in the MDS can speak for the distribution of causes of mortality in India as a whole. The answer to this question consists both of multiple mappings of Indian health made with the data and of how to relate to the specific purposes of the study. At the same time, we will see how the study's claim to representativeness is not uncontested.

Analysts of statistics and other quantified measures of the world have long observed how numbers bring things into being (Porter, 1996; Espeland & Stevens, 2008). To count things is to turn them into objects of both knowledge and governance, creating not only the quantified objects themselves, but also (state) institutions that have authority over these numbers as well as, for instance, groups of citizens and their rights and responsibilities (Saetnan et al., 2011). In the domain of (global health) epidemiology, numerical evidence is thus attributed a certain authority in defining disease and in creating new forms of subjectivity, social groupings etc. that emerge from how health and disease are defined and classified at a collective level (Adams, 2013; Sangaramoorthy & Benton, 2012; Lorway & Khan, 2014). The question what causes of death are common in India thus has implications for how India is perceived and how priorities in health policy-making are formulated.

On the basis of MDS mortality statistics, in interviews researchers would both describe India in terms of its overall health status and on the basis of regional differences. On the one hand, researchers would list several findings from the study they found surprising or remarkable when prompted. They would for example present relatively low-profile causes of death such as road accidents and death from snake bites as more common than previously estimated, whereas HIV, for example, had a lesser impact. Malaria, to which we will return later, was found to be more common than expected, as was death from smoking related disease, despite lower tobacco consumption and later ages at which people in India started smoking. To explain this, one researcher formulated the hypothesis of a link between smoking deaths and tuberculosis, which is still widespread in India.

Zooming out from individual findings, however, study personnel would point to the so-called epidemiological transition as a key dimension of public health in India (Rajan & Prabhakaran, 2012). As one of the study's initiators explained:

> The burden of disease in India and many developing countries is shifting. You have an economic transition and in the Million Death Study data you see that not only infectious diseases are prominent in India, but there are many chronic diseases that are emerging.

At the same time, this transition from infectious to chronic or non-communicable diseases as predominant causes of death is considered to be still ongoing and incomplete in India. A different researcher thus emphasized the "residual burden" of infectious disease and argued that this manifested, for example, in "India [having] a unique blend of deaths from heart attacks at premature ages, which has global relevance for prevention". Here, it is worth noting both how "India" takes on specific significance in terms of its intermediary epidemiological status and how my respondent emphasized the relevance of this fact for *(global)* disease prevention.

Interview respondents would not only talk about India's overall epidemiological status, though, but would also highlight how the MDS provides insight into regional differences. The study manual, for example, lists regional differences in common diseases and the factors contributing to them as one of the issues the study focuses on (SRS Collaborators of the RGI-CGHR, 2011). Bringing the interest in regional differences to a point, one researcher told me how "each common disease is rare somewhere in India. So, it is rare here, we can avoid this thing"—again establishing a specific link between MDS findings and disease prevention. Elaborating on this statement, he further placed India in a broader global health context by observing how the country has a "huge population, and diverse, which reflects the whole developing world". Along these lines, he argued that some of the most striking differences could be found between (richer) Southern states and what he described as the Hindu heartland, suggesting that "development" was a major factor by which differences could be explained, even though "we have not gathered data on the reasons for differences". His discussion of regional differences thereby resonates both with observations about the way mapping of disease distributions forms "a way of making sense of health and disease in populations in the world" (Koch, 2017, p. 6) and the way maps may symbolically represent certain territories and their significance (Anderson, 2006). At the same time, regional mappings of disease prevalence contributes to the "legibility" (Scott, 1999) of disease in terms of both making health problems visible and intervening in them.

At the same time, the established grid of geographical classification of Indian states clashes with the desired degree of precision of the MDS to show some of the latter's statistical limitations. Study results are not very meaningful at the level of certain smaller states. One interview respondent illustrated this by saying, "if you go to Goa, for a lot of diseases it is too small and they have a lot of fluctuation [in findings compared year-to-year]". As this quote suggests, this issue is distinct relative to the specific prevalence of diseases. Thus, two researchers I interviewed jointly explained the issue by one of them pointing out how "cancer can be reasonably captured at the national level and largely, if not for the states, for the zones at least[2]". To this, his colleague added: "if you go for colon cancer it is difficult, because it is such a rare disease. Now, if you go for breast cancer you might get a good estimate". Yet this is not only an issue in terms of capturing a sufficient number of cases of a certain cause of death as a function of state size. It is most of all a product of how SRS sampling leads to "an undercount in vital rates".

However, as the researcher flagging this problem explained further, the issue is considered relatively minor, based on the assumption that deaths missed in the sample are largely similar to those included. He considers this assumption "fair", by observing how the distribution of missing deaths is "kind of random" and not clustered geographically or by age. Moreover, he again contrasted the MDS with the alternative, which would be to rely on hospital-based statistics. Illustrating the shortcomings of these statistics he pointed out how "[p]eople who go to hospitals and die are very different from those who stay home and die [...] If you base the national estimates on hospital statistics, you get really misleading numbers". Clinical statistics are not sufficiently representative, and even though MDS statistics are not a "gold standard", the argument is that they provide better and more useful mappings of causes of death in India than hospital statistics do.

The idea that MDS statistics are not only more accurate but also more useful forms another key aspect of the confidence researchers have in the study's significance for public health in India in spite of its limitations. As observers of global health metrics and evidence based medicine have noted, the presumption that decontextualized data provides direct evidence of which health problems matter in which ways is strongly linked to ideas about the specific kinds of interventions that are most likely to succeed—even if important aspects of health and disease are thereby blended out (Bell, 2017; Adams, 2016). Such presumptions are strongly present in interview respondents' explanations of reasons for establishing the MDS. One researcher referred to its "policy impact" multiple times during our conversation. Another one argued that "the first thing" in establishing the study was to "[produce] data for advocacy purposes [...] changing the mindset of the administrators". This line of thinking is, for example, also reflected in a proposal for a new approach to health policy and health care coverage in India co-authored by MDS-director Prabhat Jha (Jha & Laxminarayan, 2009). A core part of this proposal is to expand health care coverage by providing tailored services focused on the most pressing health issues in India, as identified through cause of death data.

In another attempt to make clear how the Million Death Study has an impact, one researcher referred to the aforementioned numbers of people dying from snakebites. He illustrated the scale of the problem by citing a number of around 5000 deaths found in the study, which is vastly higher than the number of 900 found in what he described as government statistics (see also Mohapatra et al., 2011). As he continued to explain, "snakebites are happening at home, so nobody knows. So, now the government has changed their policies. The anti-venom availability [...]. We showed how in the monsoon time it is happening more. So all these things we analyse". This person thereby articulated a widespread belief among MDS staff: that the main value of their data lies in allowing more appropriate health interventions.

However, the Million Death Study does not only find that certain ICD-codes are more likely to cause deaths in India than others. Lack of availability and accessibility of medical care as well as other social factors emerge as major health problems from the data as well. As the same researcher illustrated:

> So, this is a particular village, and your hospital is fifteen kilometres away. So reaching the hospital is a problem. And if the hospital is there, the doctor might not be available. If the doctor is available, facilities may not be available.

On the surface, such a finding is not surprising. Both the link of deficient social institutions and social inequalities to mortality and the importance of social causes of disease are well established in health research (Hertzman & Siddiqi, 2009; Cockerham, 2013). Yet even when considering social determinants of health, there is often a tendency to reduce them to measurable, singular "factors" that obscure the complex relational and constantly changing practices of health and disease (Yates-Doerr, 2020). For public health in India, this raises real concerns that complex dimensions of mortality that are not included in a narrowly conceived medical domain may not be sufficiently considered in health policy (Rao et al., 2015).

One MDS researcher seemed to suggest that wider social inequalities affect mortality data collection, too, when describing "some weaknesses in the verbal autopsy". As he described it, VA

> is based on the experience of the caregiver, so he [sic!] gives the information. Some people are well educated, some people are poor, illiterate guys. So there are some doubts about the narrative details sometimes.

And yet, he insisted, out of multiple causes of death (co-morbidity), only one is registered in the hospital as well. Moreover, he concluded, "there is no alternative [to the MDS] for India. In the immediate future, there will not be clinically certified deaths in India".[3] In spite of its diagnostic shortcomings, the MDS is thus seen as the best thing available at this point.

Shortcomings in diagnostic outcomes and mortality statistics are therefore evaluated against this background, leading to understandings of disease burdens that echo the use of equivalent codes in assigning individual causes of death. Using the examples of ICD-codes J44 and J45, which describe asthma and chronic obstructive pulmonary disease (COPD), respectively, one researcher indicated how:

> even though they are separate elements, if I correlate, say 44 and [my colleague] has 45, the system takes it as equivalent cause. Etiologically they may be different, but as far as the burden of disease is concerned, it makes hardly any difference.

A different respondent argued in a similar vein, claiming that "a lot of the time you don't have to get the exact medical diagnosis". He continued to explain how often, VA does not allow for differentiation at the most exact level. Yet, he also stated how "this stratification is not required from the population point of view. [...] VA is very good from the public health intervention point of view. [...] That is the strength of the project." Not only does MDS data allow for more accurate interventions (which, to put a bow on it, would largely be the same ones for both asthma and COPD), it also uses "the representative strength of SRS", which raises "the possibility of being representative of the Indian population". Even if this may in certain cases lead to a loss of diagnostic specificity, so one researcher argued, "because of this, this is a reasonable estimate we have got. And whether cancer is more important than something else". The representative value of the MDS and what that allows for in terms of public health interventions is thus considered more valuable than diagnostic precision.

Still, some commentators focus exactly on the question of diagnostic accuracy in scrutinizing the study. One article that seeks to link the study to the United Nation's Millenium Development Goals by asking whether the former can help in monitoring the latter (Bhutta, 2006) raises some questions about the adequacy of the SRS for making statistically significant statements about cause-specific infant death, among other issues. As indicated above, this is an issue that MDS researchers recognize and for which they do, for example, present findings at a higher level of temporal or geographical aggregation. More troubling, at least for MDS personnel,[4] is an article in *Nature* that questioned the verbal autopsy method, specifically on the basis of the study's findings on malaria deaths (Butler, 2010). The article suggested that the far higher number of deaths attributed to malaria in the MDS than are counted in the government's malaria control programme result from an overestimation. This, in turn, is said to be due to biases coding physicians bring to the interpretation of symptomatic data, in particular by assuming that fever syndromes are probably malaria. While there is widespread agreement that official statistics underestimate malaria and although MDS results show the same distribution of malaria in India as the control programme does (see, e.g., Dhingra et al., 2010), the *Nature* article thus presumes the latter's errors to not be quite as egregious as MDS data suggests.

When I confronted MDS-researchers with this article in interviews (which they—of course—all knew already), they mostly took it as an opportunity to once more explain the value of the study. Almost all of them made a version of the claim that they "are not saying that this is a gold standard for malaria deaths". Most pointed out that a certain diagnosis of malaria requires microbiological confirmation. Instead, so one of them told me, the study works with "a history that there is an adult who had an acute fever and dropped dead". Yet he continued to argue that a malaria diagnosis would be reasonable in such a case since,

> you have to think logically. There aren't that many things [that may cause such a scenario] in the geographic distributions where those occur. So it's probably true that there might be some other things, dengue, or others going on. But it is also true that some of the deaths we call dengue or pneumonia are actually malaria. Misclassification works both ways[5].

Furthermore, he pointed out once more how MDS findings map exactly onto the distribution of confirmed cases.

Another respondent compared the malaria control programme's reliance on microbiologically confirmed malaria deaths to the "symptomatic" definition used by the MDS. Expanding on this contrast, he explained how only people diagnosed in a clinical setting would be included in the official numbers. What he described as "non-users" of government services would thus be overlooked, whereas the MDS, "we are going to households. So we are encompassing the whole population. We accept that the operational definitions differ. But they are not getting any numbers on non-users". What this means, for example (or so another researcher indicated), is that MDS data on mortality from malaria shows a U-shaped age distribution of deaths, which suggests that the disease is more likely to be lethal for people more vulnerable due to low or high age. The suggestion here seems to be that the MDS does not only allow more representative, but also more fine-grained insight into the distribution of causes of death.

Finally, a third argument in response to this article revolved once more around the question how important diagnostic accuracy is beyond a certain threshold. As one person I interviewed who had made the switch from research to health programme administration said, "for a program implementer it is more important—do the same study after a few years and see what happens [...] You use a methodology, ten years down the line you use the same methodology and tell us the results". As indicated by another researcher, such a longer term perspective can show if policy interventions have had any effects, since the results show up in SRS and MDS data.

In response to a controversy that emerged around the specific mortality attributed to malaria, people involved with the MDS thus once more reiterated that the true value of the study lies in its implications for health policy making, its inclusion of representative, non-clinical data and the way it allows reasonable diagnosis even in the absence of clinical certification (which is not available for the majority of deaths in India). While this may not result in diagnoses that accord to a scientific gold standard, it does supposedly produce more *practically reliable* insight into nationwide mortality. In sum, the controversy over malaria numbers vividly illustrates the multiple meanings of mortality data, which can be both accurate and inaccurate at the same time, depending on the form of accuracy one prioritizes.

It would, however, be a mistake to only see the MDS as a vehicle for improving health policy-making in India. The study also contains scientific ambitions and these extend beyond India, too. Thus, one researcher maintains that a key insight from the study is that "if you get a random sample of deaths—and that's the key, it's a true random sample, you can't just go to the hospital—you get a really good snapshot of what is going on". Such a snapshot, so various people suggested, might also be generated for other low- and middle-income countries without sufficient certified mortality statistics by using the same method. This is not least due to the diversity of India, which is sometimes interpreted to mean that the country is itself a kind of sample for the global South at large. One premier researcher links this perception of the study to a broader global health imaginary. Implicitly referencing the Sustainable Development Goals, this person mused how "we have examples of these global efforts and I think another simple one is: count the dead by 2030. That every country has some information from a random sample of how its people die".

Beyond this role as a global exemplar, various researchers also described the MDS as a "hypothesis-generating study" or a "platform for discovery", suggesting that "more specific studies" to, for example, find out what causes the prevalence of certain causes of death could be developed. The MDS thereby also serves as a research infrastructure in the sense of what Slota and Bowker (2017) describe in terms of work done to enable other kinds of work.

The development of the verbal autopsy method and its proposed utility beyond India further complicate any straightforward notions of a narrative emphasizing the deficiency of the Indian state in the context of public health. As many scholars focusing on science, medicine and public health in (post)colonial India have observed, imperialist marginalization of population health has left significant traces, but cannot fully account for contemporary relations between science and the state (Seth, 2009; Phalkey, 2013). While MDS researchers would thus reference the remnants of British bureaucracy as a key factor hindering certified mortality administration or the dual disease burden in terms of stunted economic development, the study itself may be seen as an innovative way of generating mortality statistics and redefining the state's responsibility in the process. Put differently, without denying the shadows of (post)colonialism in the troubled status of public health in India (Kumar, 2001; Palit, 2005), the MDS also invites us to question sedimented discourses and "imaginative geographies" of postcolonial health sciences (Prasad, 2014b, 2016). Suggesting an alternative view of science in India, Itty Abraham (2006, p. 217) proposes "leaves the cartographic map unsettled as the presumed stable geopolitical entity called 'India' is called into account in different ways". The case of the MDS says that the map of India's population can be similarly unsettled, being assembled, disassembled and reassembled not only to provide evidence of causes of death, but also to pursue innovative ways of doing data-based population research.

Conclusion: Reassembling Population in the Production of Mortality Statistics

The Million Death Study in India formed a response to an alleged deficit in knowledge about the most common causes of death in the country, which was in turn seen as a major shortcoming for public health. Study initiators therefore developed an alternative way of mapping population health that could function independently of medically certified mortality statistics, which were considered inaccurate and inadequate (see Fig. 4.1 for the study procedure).

To this end, the MDS built on an existing infrastructure for constructing statistics on population dynamics, the Sample Registration System, which was in itself a tool for gaining insight into population changes during the 10-year intervals of the full census. Through its dual enumeration structure, the SRS created a particular version of India's population, to which a data collection method called verbal autopsy was added. Verbal autopsy relied on an assumption that disease symptoms would be pronounced just prior to a person's death, thus allowing their description and registration by medical laypersons. As such, symptomatic data was considered to be free of premature interpretation. Yet for interpretation, a combination of medically trained 'coders', a refined diagnostic procedure and electronic decision support were supposed to generate accurate diagnosis—at least at a (limited) level of precision adequate for public health. These individual diagnoses would then be aggregated into both national and—depending on the prevalence of a condition—specific subnational mortality statistics, which, again, could have a lesser degree of precision if this could be considered acceptable from a public health perspective. Consequently, the MDS aims to produce more accurate and representative insight into population health that could inform public

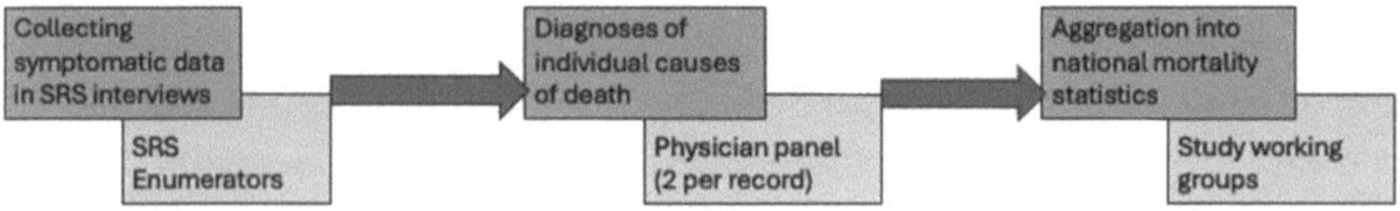

Fig. 4.1 Data collection and analysis procedure of the Million Death Study

health policy—or, in the words of one interview respondent, insights that "contribute to corrections in assumptions and changes in priorities".

This characterization of the study begs the question which assumptions and priorities the MDS itself contains. As we have seen throughout this chapter, it heavily relies on a combination of critique of state-based health monitoring infrastructures and the use of alternative state infrastructures to generate and process alternative data. This paradoxical questioning of and reliance on the state generates a particular perspective on population and population health within the study. Most significantly, population health comes to be rendered in technical, diagnostic terms that the study manual itself characterizes as a "one-death-one cause situation" (SRS Collaborators of the RGI-CGHR, 2011, p. 9). To be sure, this approach has great value. It circumvents some of the limitations of relying on clinical diagnosis only, which study researchers—I think convincingly—consider wholly inadequate for India because it misses large parts of the (especially rural) population and the vastly different causes of deaths that occur without medical attention.

Yet, I would also draw on Arturo Escobar's (2011) critique of the entanglements of knowledge and power in development discourse by acknowledging how "[s]tatistics tell stories [and] are techno-representations endowed with complex political and cultural histories". In the case of the MDS, these histories are not only linked to the colonial roots of India's deficiencies in public health, but also the sociotechnical apparatus of global health and its emphasis on decontextualized statistical evidence in developing both measurements of and interventions in population health in the Global South (Reubi, 2018; Birn, 2009; Adams, 2016). Against this background, we may conceive of the MDS as an infrastructure for the purpose of *population-based* medical research that creates its population base in a specific statistical form that maps it as an aggregate of both national and regionally distinct causes of death with probable significance for other countries 'like' India. Yet as statistics tend to do, they exclude many aspects of what makes a population, not least of them the idea of a demos that might have a voice expressing more than stories registered for the purpose of distilling symptomatic data points. This specific understanding of health data thus renders a relatively narrow understanding of population.

Within the Million Death Study, we thus see how a population is rendered as multiple (Mol, 2003) across several axes that all, in one way or another, are related to data. On the one hand, there is the simultaneous move towards more accurate data and acceptance of a degree of inaccuracy in light of the study's purpose. On the other hand the collection of mortality data through verbal autopsy is simultaneously a project in critique of the state's knowledge infrastructures and one relying on 'the state'. What the state and its role in contemporary public health is, is thereby continuously negotiated. Finally, the population is itself made multiple through various forms of data. It is a set of individuals with symptoms as much as a national unit in the middle of an epidemiological transition, as well as a collection of socioeconomically distinct regional populations that stand in for low- and middle-income countries in general. Such questions of data accuracy and the relation between state and other actors are not unique to the Million Death Study (Singh, 2019), nor, presumably, to India. Delving into how the Million Death Study makes population by making data, and back, thus provide particular insight into population-based medical research in the age of 'big data'.

The reference to big data approaches in research, as well as the particular relation between existing state infrastructures and the involvement of global health institutions, suggests that medical research is multifaceted in the Million Death Study. How medical research may then also come to mean different, and occasionally conflicting, things is an issue we explore further in the next chapter, where we turn our attention back to genomic biobanking, and to Europe.

Notes

1. See https://cghr-toronto.github.io/va-course/course/data/video1.mp4 (last accessed 9 July 2025).
2. Zones in India are more expansive geographical units that include a number of states. India is divided into six such zones in which states are expected to cooperate on certain issues.

3. There are, of course, but by now it should be well established that a central article of faith for the MDS is that these are neither accurate (in most cases) nor representative of India's population as a whole.
4. While I will turn to researchers' substantive arguments against the claims brought forward in the article next, I would be amiss not to mention one respondent describing this piece of writing with a somewhat more colloquial term for equine manure.
5. Not only does misclassification work both ways, so another researcher suggested, but for vector-borne diseases such as malaria and dengue it is also immaterial what the exact diagnosis is, since the required preventive interventions would be roughly the same.

5

Disputing Medical Research in the European Research Infrastructure BBMRI-ERIC

In May 2020, during the early months of the COVID-19 pandemic when most public events had moved online, I virtually attended a conference titled "*European Research Infrastructures for a smarter future*".[1] The conference was jointly organized by Croatia, holding the rotating European Union (EU) presidency at the time, and the European Strategy Forum for Research Infrastructure (ESFRI), an intergovernmental EU body. As a sign of the times, the question how Europe would manage the pandemic in the present and recover from its effects in the future received central attention. The diverse range of speakers from research and policy institutions largely agreed that European research infrastructures had to play a central role on both counts. Antonio Andreu, the scientific director of EATRIS, the European research infrastructure for translational medicine, for example, contributed his reflections on the importance of research infrastructures in the context of COVID-19 to a panel discussion. Andreu argued on behalf of several biomedical research infrastructures[2] that they play key roles in improving quality, reproducibility and cooperation in research. Research infrastructures thereby pursue "stable cross-border collaboration [as] the way forward". In that sense, he maintained, "COVID is a perfect challenge in building Europe". He thereby at once reproduced a rhetorical trope that sees European integration as

E. Aarden, *Producing Citizenship in Medical Research Collections*, Health, Technology and Society, https://doi.org/10.1007/978-981-95-1707-7_5

critical in responding to existential crises, and placed research infrastructures squarely at the heart of European integration efforts. More central to my purpose in this chapter, his particular representation of biomedical research infrastructures suggested that 'medical research' can do and be multiple different things at the same time. This left me wondering: When looking at such (European) infrastructures for the purpose of (population-based) medical research, what does the label *medical research* stand for?

This question is at the centre of this chapter, where I explore the European Biobanking and Biomolecular Resources Research Infrastructure–European Research Infrastructure Consortium (BBMRI-ERIC for short and from here on out). Understanding this infrastructure as a product of European Union (EU) science policy, I am particularly interested in how various dimensions of medical research practice and organization are brought together, but also into conflict, in this infrastructure. A central idea behind this infrastructure is that both the scientific and social value of research can be enhanced through networking, i.e., by making stored materials and data accessible to geographically and institutionally distributed researchers (Mayrhofer et al., 2016; Langhof et al., 2017). BBMRI-ERIC itself thus emphasizes in one of its annual Work Programmes how its "ultimate goal" is "to facilitate access to biological resources as well as biomedical facilities and to support high-quality biomolecular and medical research" (BBMRI-ERIC, 2015b, p. 3). In this case, "infrastructuring" is thereby presented as a central element of medical research.

By facilitating access to materials stored in tissue and data repositories around Europe, BBMRI-ERIC is expected to contribute to different aspects of what medical research can (supposedly) be. It forms a network of so-called biobanks, or collections of tissue and medical data created for research (Parodi, 2015; Kinkorová, 2016). Biobanks supposedly contribute value for translational research (Murtagh et al., 2011), epidemiology (Zielhuis, 2012), biomarker research (Végvári et al., 2011) and better healthcare (Riegman et al., 2008)—to present just a (small) sample of research promises made around biobanking. However, in line with the supposedly growing scale of medical research (see also Chaps. 2 and 3), single biobanks are increasingly considered too small for answering medicine's most pressing questions. Biobank promoters therefore argue that larger datasets generated through merging, pooling or exchanging between existing collections are required (Asslaber & Zatloukal, 2007; Shickle & Griffin, 2009; Simell et al., 2019). According to the Business Plan for BBMRI-ERIC, this European network can meet such requirements. Arguments for such a European endeavour include its value for enabling the study of "important biomedical research questions that are beyond the scope of efforts of single Member States[3]" to thereby "reduce fragmentation of the European research landscape and [increase] competitiveness through collaboration". In this focus on collaboration and competitiveness, then, the label 'medical research' is already doing different kinds of work in the planning for BBMRI-ERIC (Zatloukal et al., 2012, p. 11).

It is noteworthy here how the challenge of research questions requiring large databases is intricately woven together with ideas of European collaboration and competitiveness (see also Lauss, 2009). Along similar lines, BBMRI-ERIC's first Director General (DG) Jan-Eric Litton (2018, p. 240) argued a few years later how the infrastructure is "unique", thus "giving Europe a striking competitive advantage" that should make it possible to "harvest [biobanks'] benefits for European citizens in the future". Moreover, so one interview respondent as well as several publications emphasized, this resource is readily available, since "we have a hundred million samples in those banks in Europe, they are waiting to be used". The rhetoric surrounding BBMRI-ERIC builds on the general value of such collections for large-scale research that can be productive in various ways. Yet it also emphasizes the specific advantages Europe supposedly already has in this domain and can capitalize on through extended collaboration.

Research in this context is thus characterized in terms of the ability to answer certain questions, but also in terms of competitiveness, generating future benefits and European collaboration. My aim in this chapter is not to define what medical research really means or to diagnose any sort of corruption to science as an epistemic enterprise by any other purposes it purportedly serves. Rather, I see the exercise in this chapter in terms akin to STS research on what science is claimed (not) to be in particular settings. This approach has perhaps been most influentially elaborated in Thomas Gieryn's (1995, 1999) notion of boundary work. Gieryn distinguishes between "[e]ssentialists [who] do boundary work [and] constructivists who watch it get done by people in society" (Gieryn, 1995, p. 394).

Science, then, can be seen as a marker that is "empty *until* its insides get filled and its borders drawn amidst context-bound negotiations over who and what is "scientific"" (Gieryn, 1995, p. 405). Boundary work, for Gieryn, is about struggles over cognitive authority and other resources associated with an activity or claim being recognized as "scientific". While I do not so much focus on the drawing of boundaries between science and non-science, I find Gieryn's approach helpful in tracing what the notion of science (or most commonly research, which I will loosely define as 'doing science' and use interchangeably) *does* in claims regarding the benefits and shortcomings of BBMRI-ERIC.

Similar to Gieryn's observation that "the 'essential features' of science are provisional and contextual *results* of who wins" (Gieryn, 1995, p. 406), claims surrounding BBMRI-ERIC's importance for medical research must be read within a broader context of the shifting social status and significance of science over the last few decades. David Guston (2000) has observed how, since the middle of the twentieth century, science policy has shifted from a "social contract" of presumed productivity to increasingly explicit political expectations of and efforts to exercise control over the presumed productivity of research. Exploring what such shifts (may) mean for scientific research, other observers have proposed notions like the Triple Helix (Etzkowitz, 2008), post-normal science (Funtowicz & Ravetz, 1993) or Mode-2 science (Gibbons et al., 1994) to each highlight different aspects of the tightening entanglements and increased complexity of relations between science, society, industry and politics. More specifically targeted at the life sciences, a further strand of literature has focused on the question if and how expectations of economic productivity, commodification and speculation affect research and innovation (Sunder Rajan, 2006; Cooper, 2008; Birch & Tyfield, 2013; Chiapetta & Birch, 2018). Finally, in the particular European context, "[f]rom its very inception European Union knowledge politics were interwoven in the complex game of European integration" (Benner, 2018, p. 117). Investments in research have become increasingly integral to the European integration process, intersecting both with efforts at European state-building and promoting economic competitiveness.

Against this background of shifting science-society relations and science's advancing role in European integration, this chapter touches upon questions relevant beyond the case of BBMRI-ERIC or the domain of medical research infrastructures. Research infrastructures as such have become increasingly prominent in science policy in Europe (and beyond), although the vast variety of configurations established under this heading in different disciplines raises questions about its conceptual significance (Cramer et al., 2020). One thing research infrastructures do, however, is to link broader organizational and political frameworks to scientific work, particularly through the production of shared standards (Duclos Lindstrøm & Kropp, 2017). Moving from research infrastructures and science policy to other domains of EU activity, standardization is a central element in creating what Andrew Barry (2001, 2006) describes as a "technological zone", a sphere of governance in which technical arrangements set the rules of engagement (see also Dunn, 2005). As we will see in the case of BBMRI-ERIC, such technological zones are not uncontested and have significance beyond the aim to harmonize specific domains of (scientific) work. This, in turn, affects how this medical research infrastructure is imagined to serve a European population that is itself conjured as a product of building the infrastructure.

Making European Science Through Research Infrastructures

The establishment of BBMRI-ERIC resulted from a lengthy development process initiated and shaped by a move in EU science policy towards building research infrastructures. Yet the reasons for BBMRI (as it was initially called) to be among the first formally recognized European research infrastructures include the aforementioned rising need for large data and sample collections in research. The infrastructure's business plan lists three motivations for its establishment: Europe's aging population, the need to understand genetic and environmental causes of disease, as well as the need to "translate" such new knowledge into treatments provide the main motivations for efforts to interconnect European biobanks (Zatloukal et al., 2012). The required scale of data and samples, so a group of authors involved in the early set-up of BBMRI has further argued, can only be achieved in a federated network established in different countries (Yuille et al., 2007). It should therefore not be too surprising that political efforts to build cross-national institutional collaborations for science, or "research infrastructures" as these were increasingly called, aligned very well with such scientific ambitions—even though, so one respondent involved in this early phase told me, large-scale infrastructure was a novel phenomenon in the domain of biomedical research.

The desire to interlink medical tissue and data collections received a particular impulse from the establishment of the European Strategy Forum for Research Infrastructures (ESFRI) at the beginning of this century. As Jan-Eric Litton, BBMRI-ERIC's first Director General explained to me, ESFRI was "the [EU] Member States who got together. And they really wanted to build infrastructure for Europe". This idea, he continued, was then picked up by the European Commission, which supported the development of a first ESFRI Roadmap in 2006, which included a list of research infrastructures prioritized for development and implementation (European Strategy Forum on Research Infrastructures, 2006). Among the prioritized infrastructures was a network of biobanks that, so one person described, had as one of its main goals to "develop [a] process how to access several biobanks in parallel" and in spite of cross-national differences in legislation and access procedures. The development of this network, as well as of several other early research infrastructures, received further support in the form of project funding under the European Commission's seventh framework programme. This project for biobanking became known as the BBMRI preparatory phase. It ran from 2007 until 2011 with the aim to develop an outline or blueprint for this research infrastructure.

The project was organized into different work packages that largely trace the organizational structure of BBMRI-ERIC as it exists today and had the business plan as its major output. However, in the meantime the European Commission had taken further steps in formalizing research infrastructures as a science policy instrument by introducing the ERIC legal framework. ERIC, which stands for European Research Infrastructure Consortium, gives formal legal recognition to cross-national research infrastructures under European law. Such infrastructures are framed as collaborative entities based on membership of individual countries, at least half of which also need to be EU members. This legal entity was introduced to further advance European science, both by simplifying the coordination between (primarily) EU member states and by stimulating further scientific collaboration (Moskovko et al., 2019). Yet, as a generic legal format balancing the interests of the European community with those of individual member states in the regulation and implementation of scientific collaboration, ERIC is restricted in terms of what it prescribes for harmonization issues in specific scientific disciplines (Reichel, 2015). Former Director-General Jan-Eric Litton, for example, told me how the general legal formation of ERIC "doesn't care anything about [...] sharing samples across borders". As it became increasingly clear throughout the preparatory phase that the ERIC legal format would be applied to BBMRI, this lack of specificity would create some lasting effects.

Former Director-General Jan-Eric Litton suggests that the relatively limited relevance of the ERIC regulation also created problems in moving from the preparatory phase to a more sustainable status. He described the time between the end of the preparatory phase in 2011 and formal recognition of BBMRI-ERIC in 2013 as "the dead period", arguing that much time was lost on "the political things". These included several areas that required agreement between the member states, including the choice for a particular governance model and how to finance the infrastructure. The membership model that was ultimately chosen, which I will discuss in-depth below, is nevertheless seen positively by several interview respondents, particularly in terms of the relative ease by which member states can join, regardless of size and existing (national) biobanking infrastructure.

While BBMRI-ERIC has thus formally been recognized as a European research infrastructure since 2013, its implementation has been supported by a further project with Framework Programme funding. In the context of the Horizon 2020 funding programme, BBMRI-ERIC ran the ADOPT-BBMRI project between 2015 and 2018. This project, as described in BBMRI-ERIC's 2015 Annual Report was aimed at "boosting and accelerating implementation of BBMRI-ERIC and its services" (BBMRI-ERIC, 2016a, p. 90). To do so, the project included work packages aimed at enhancing several of the biobanking services (including in the fields of Ethical, Legal and Social Issues (ELSI), information technology (IT) and quality management), as well as an effort to build a cohort for studying colorectal cancer from the collections of member biobanks.

Within the project, implementation efforts hence focused on facilitating access to available materials, reducing fragmentation of the research landscape and capacity building in countries with less developed biobanking communities (BBMRI-ERIC, 2017c). In the eyes of BBMRI-ERIC staff member Lukasz Kozera, the latter is an important aspect, since there are significant differences between member states also in terms of the treatment patients receive. He therefore explained how "obviously, countries like Austria and Belgium, which are really well developed when it comes to medical care, they will provide a different diagnostic or treatment facility comparing for example to Poland or Lithuania". Work to harmonize certain aspects of research, he thus suggests, may also help in harmonizing medical care. From a perhaps more critical perspective, French biobanker Georges Dagher describes ADOPT as not a scientific project, but as building a database. Building a database as part of a project is one specific example of the "infrastructuring" of European research that happens throughout the development and operation of BBMRI-ERIC (Aarden, 2023), a process that may also be summarized as "a materialization of the process of European integration" (Lauss, 2009, p. 265).

This emphasis on research infrastructures in EU science policy reflects how the EU has "positioned science and technology as vanguards of political and social integration" (Trischler & Kohlrausch, 2014, p. 280). Yet various historians have observed how process of European integration through science and technology have not exclusively or necessarily been linked to the formal integration project of the EU (Papon, 2004; Hallonsten, 2012). Not only is the "project" of the EU itself far from linear and straightforward (Patel, 2018), European integration has always—or at least since large cross-border infrastructure building in the nineteenth century—"depended on and was shaped by material networks, technical systems, and the circulation of knowledge and artifacts" (Misa & Schot, 2005, p. 2). Historians of technology therefore argue for decentralizing the formal, political European integration process, focusing instead of processes of hidden integration (Kaiser & Schot, 2014; Misa & Schot, 2005; Schipper & Schot, 2011). Here, "in many ways, technological infrastructures are indeed the essence of European integration" (Badenoch & Fickers, 2010, p. 2). More specific to BBMRI-ERIC,

European integration can take the form of building a material infrastructure and implementing European policy *simultaneously*.

The notion of research infrastructure is presently quite prominent in EU research policy. But, in line with historical work on 'hidden integration' the making of transnational 'European' scientific institutions long predates the processes of economic and political collaboration that ultimately resulted in the EU. The first large facilities were established in the 1950s, with distributed facilities emerging from the 1980s onwards (Papon, 2004). Although such collaborations were historically detached from European integration processes, they were characterized by similar tensions between national sovereignty and ideas of a shared European common good (Hallonsten, 2012). The recent emphasis on European research infrastructures is simultaneously claimed to be void of significance, since it remains unclear what the notion entails across its many different forms (Hallonsten, 2020). At the same time, and beyond science and innovation, what it means to be European is equally uncertain and contested (Pagden, 2002). Different entities and institutions get defined as 'European' in conjunction with the various meanings and purposes attributed to research and research infrastructures.

Nevertheless, the notion of research infrastructures does have significance for understanding the multiple identities of (medical) research in transnational science policy in Europe. In the case of BBMRI-ERIC for example, it seems significant that part of what defines it as an infrastructure is that it is not a project. One of the infrastructure's Work Programme's further explores the differences in terms of how, as a research infrastructure, "it is not about finalizing deliverables and reaching milestones, but about building and implementing sustainable services for the European biobank and biomolecular resources community" (BBMRI-ERIC, 2016d, p. 2). What makes an infrastructure thus seems to be sustainable service delivery; however, this does not seem to be possible without implementation projects. Both the aforementioned ADOPT project and the Large Population Cohorts (LPC) projects that bridged the period between the preparatory phase and ERIC status had a vital function in implementing BBMRI-ERIC.

The LPC project was aimed at "[exploring] facilitated transnational access to samples and data" (BBMRI-ERIC, 2016b, p. 10) and developing" 'best practices' for transnational access" (BBMRI-ERIC, 2016b, p. 11). Preparatory phase coordinator Eero Vuorio described this in an interview as "essentially a test of how BBMRI-ERIC actually works", a characterization echoed in another person's description of the ADOPT project as a transition from "construction" to "operation". Here, the key task was supposedly that "we must show that we can do biobanking". Beyond these two implementation projects, BBMRI-ERIC further also continues to be a participant in European research projects, a practice that is not uncontroversial, since some people believe that, as a European research infrastructure, it should be a facilitator of medical research projects and not a participant in them. Such controversy thus shows how it is not straightforward what medical research means, or what the role of infrastructures in such research is.

Things get even more complicated when considering how BBMRI-ERIC was set up to be a European research infrastructure. Both the labels European and research are contested and get continuously negotiated—not least in relation to each other. Almost from the beginning, the construction that was to be BBMRI-ERIC has been characterized as "best described as a distributed hub structure" (Yuille et al., 2007, p. 16). This description refers to how individual biobanks are members of BBMRI-ERIC only indirectly, via national hubs. Particularly under the conditions set by the ERIC framework, national states are the actual members of BBMRI-ERIC. This has created a somewhat complex, multi-layered governance structure. As one person involved in managing the preparatory phase describes it,

> [t]here are not the individual biobanks part of BBMRI, but it's the, it's always a national network of biobanks. We wanted to have a strong national coordination in each of the countries.

Individual biobanks are thus part of so-called National Nodes, which collectively form BBMRI-ERIC (see Fig. 5.1). To coordinate activities between these national nodes and provide certain so-called "common services", BBMRI-ERIC also has an executive office, commonly known as headquarters, which—in line with the ERIC regulation—is led by a Director-General and located in Graz, in Austria, which is the infrastructure's 'host country'.[4]

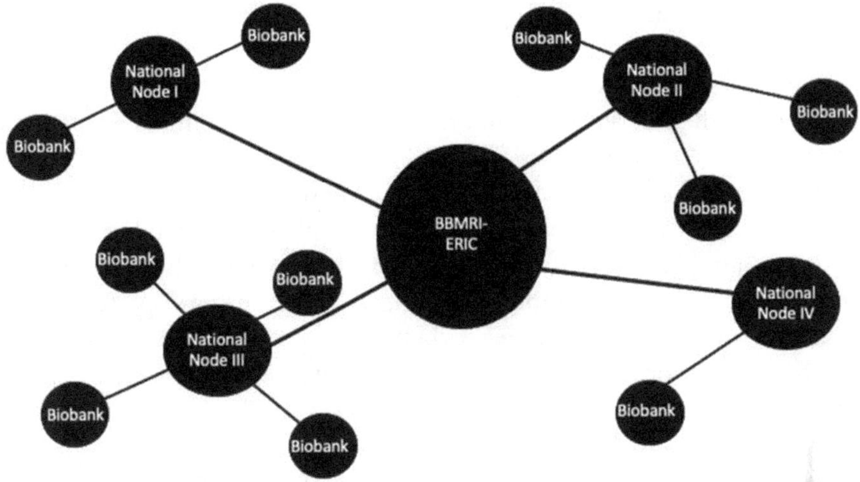

Fig. 5.1 The distributed 'hub-and-spoke' organizational structure of BBMRI-ERIC. (Figure by the author, originally published in Aarden (2023))

ERIC regulations and several official documents such as the infrastructure's Statutes and Partner Charter further define roles and responsibilities for each of the three entities (headquarters, national nodes and biobanks) that make up BBMRI-ERIC. The Director-General is appointed by the Assembly of Members. This is the infrastructure's main governing body, in which each member state is represented with one vote. Aside from full membership, so-called observer countries are not full members and also have no vote in the Assembly. The Assembly of Members also determines the annual budget, which is calculated on the basis of two categories: country size for a fixed segment, and a flexible component based on each country's GDP as a percentage of all members collective GDP (i.e., if the overall GDP of all member states would be 100 and a country has a GDP of 7, it would pay 7% of the flexible segment of BBMRI-ERIC's budget). Article 4 of the Statutes (BBMRI-ERIC, 2016c) further defines the responsibilities of member states, including tasks such as the establishment of a national node, coordinating national biobanking activities, investing in infrastructure and capacity building and implementing the infrastructure's Work Programmes. The Partner Charter (see Zatloukal et al., 2012) constitutes an agreement between the member states and individual biobanks, and commits biobanks to making samples and data available in scientific collaborations.

Member states are thus, in the words of one interview respondent, the "owners" of the infrastructure, but may not work as such in a uniform way. On the one hand, there are significant differences between member states in terms of their biobanking experience and the degree of coordination that already exists between biobanks. Preparatory phase director Eero Vuorio talked about "a North-South gradient" in biobanking in Europe, with "a tradition of collecting samples" forming a "north-of-the-Alps phenomenon". However, not only differences between countries pose a challenge for the harmonization of European biobanking within BBMRI-ERIC. As a former staff member indicated:

> there are actually two currents in BBMRI [...] the ministries, who say: we are paying, as funders we pay you for services. We want you to help biobanks in Europe. National Node directors say: you have to help me gain projects, so I can do scientific research. Those two interests, even within a country, are completely different.

Here we thus see again how interpretations of research infrastructures' meaning for medical research can differ substantially.

Cross-national differences can also affect how and to what extent the headquarters can harmonize biobanking work. While it may seem obvious that certain (cultural) differences in the area of ethics and legislation have proven difficult to resolve, collaboration has turned out not to be straightforward in other domains either. An IT-representative of one national node, for example, suggested that developing shared standards in information technology should work since "everyone speaks English and code". But national preferences in which code to use and how to distribute responsibilities for developing and running IT-systems do matter, with at least one representative of a different national node complaining to me during a conference that the Germans, who host the IT services, want to do everything their way. The so-called headquarters aims to provide a range of centralized services in the domains of ELSI, IT and quality management to address such differences—in addition to organizational coordination and project work. But centralized services need to account for the contested nature of

"Europe" and "research", too. One BBMRI-ERIC staff member thus summarized the role of the headquarters as one of balancing national and European priorities in biobanking. I'll turn to some of the practical implications of these issues next, focusing on the infrastructure's efforts in making materials accessible via IT and in quality management.

Navigating European Sample Accessibility and Quality

The question how to achieve BBMRI-ERIC's aims of sample exchange and cross-border collaboration could not be clarified by adopting the ERIC legal status alone. The infrastructure therefore required more specific rules for scientific collaboration in biobanking. Various documents that outline the structure and governance of the infrastructure include criteria for the distribution of roles within BBMRI-ERIC with regard to sample access. The Business Plan (Zatloukal et al., 2012, p. 6), for example announced that "BBMRI-ERIC will provide access to the collections of [partner biobanks], their expertise and services on a non-economic basis", while subsequently listing a number of ways how to do this. Subsequently, the plan also assured that the infrastructure "shall seek to ensure that the source of samples and data be appropriately acknowledged". These combined promises of providing access while securing acknowledgment of sample sources reflect a specific tension in the world of biobanking that is often cited as a key challenge for networking and harmonization efforts (see also Chap. 3).

Some of the ideas on how to make sure samples are made accessible outlined in the Business Plan are formalized in the BBMRI-ERIC Statutes (BBMRI-ERIC, 2016c). Article 18 focuses entirely on access and is worth quoting at length:

> BBMRI-ERIC shall make samples and data in databases affiliated with or developed by BBMRI-ERIC Partner Biobanks available to researchers and research institutions according to the access procedure and criteria as approved by the Assembly of Members. Access shall respect conditions set by sample and data providers that affiliate their databases to BBMRI-

> ERIC. No provision in these statutes should be understood as seeking to restrict the right of owners of Biobanks or Biomolecular Resources affiliated with BBMRI-ERIC to decide on providing access to any samples or data.

This description of access procedures and criteria in the Statutes remains relatively generic, but does make clear what is important to the infrastructure. On the one hand, the task of the Assembly of Members in defining access procedures and criteria is remarkable, since this body does not primarily consist of biobanking professionals but of national government representatives. The question how to access materials is thereby to some degree taken out of the context of everyday biobanking practice. At the same time, this text makes abundantly clear that even while the aim is to make materials accessible, decision making and access conditions remain in the hand of individual providers of samples and data (i.e., biobanks). Here, again, we find BBMRI-ERIC confronting the challenge of balancing interests across different layers, which resonates in the design and operation of the IT-platforms developed to facilitate access.

BBMRI-ERIC's IT platforms are intended to "ensure findability and accessibility of biobanks" (BBMRI-ERIC, 2016d, p. 3). Within this context, the infrastructure "operates as a facilitator providing access to the centrally stored data, while access to any specific samples or additional data will be granted by the partner biobanks based on their standard access procedures" (BBMRI-ERIC, 2020, p. 6). Two different platforms that function as kind of search engines form the core of the IT-infrastructure and are known as the Directory and Negotiator, respectively (Lablans et al., 2016). While the former makes it possible to find samples and data stored in member biobanks, the latter enables researchers to negotiate access to these materials.

After the Directory was launched in 2015, the Annual Report described various roles it could fill, which include making biobanks visible, identifying samples and data of interest and facilitating negotiation and access (BBMRI-ERIC, 2016a). Yet, while the claim is that the Directory "will allow biomedical and bioinformatics users to identify biobanks that might potentially have samples and/or data of interest for their research" (BBMRI-ERIC, 2015a, p. 17), the federated nature of BBMRI-ERIC makes this slightly more complex in practice. Anyone interested in samples or data can search over 500 biobanks "in bulk", as BBMRI-ERIC staff members like to say. In a webinar explaining the platform in 2019, for example, I learned how one can search for samples linked to specific diagnoses on the basis of ICD-codes. Further search criteria can then also include the type of samples, the quality of the biobank (e.g., based on accreditation) and the availability of medical records.

Based on such criteria, the Directory ideally provides a list of biobanks that fit the search criteria. Yet, I learned from the same webinar that all this depends on how disciplined biobanks are in providing the data. For example, researchers were advised not to be too specific in their search for ICD-codes, since biobanks often provide diagnostic data for samples on a more aggregate level. Furthermore, information on some search criteria is often missing or not up-to-date. In general, I learned in an interview with a BBMRI-ERIC staff member that searches in the Directory are based on aggregate statistical descriptors of the samples, including sample types, basic donor attributes, age and disease. This allows one to find biobanks that may have something relevant but does not give more detailed (clinical) data needed for research. Yet, the availability of even this basic data was seen as a challenge in the webinar. This was expressed by calling it "critical" that biobanks share what they have and want to share and thereby help each other with the visibility of individual biobanks.

Should a researcher looking for samples and data find biobanks with materials of interest in the Directory, access to these materials may be pursued with the aid of the Negotiator-platform. In a later webinar that focused exclusively on this platform, the Negotiator was described as the IT implementation of the access policy included in the BBMRI-ERIC statutes. But here, too, the "hub-and-spoke" organizational structure of the infrastructure implies that access to materials needs to be agreed with individual biobanks that hold the desired materials and data.

Contrary to the Directory, users need to authenticate before they can pose any queries in the Negotiator. The platform then allows users to pose two different kinds of requests—either a public negotiation visible to all biobanks, or a private one in which the question is posed to one specific bank. BBMRI-ERIC's executive office checks whether a query posed in the Negotiator is legitimate, but is otherwise not further involved in the negotiations. These often include a question from the addressed biobanks to specify the request for materials in return. Often, so a BBMRI-ERIC staff member informed me, researchers' initial requests are not specific enough with regard to the purposes for which materials will be used and the analytical methods applied to samples and data. Biobanks want to know these things before potentially agreeing to send out materials. If, however, researchers' requests match what a biobank is able and willing to provide, further arrangements such as material transfer agreements are made and the samples and/or data shared.

Since biobanks need to supply and maintain information about their collections for these platforms to work, lacks and lags in this information are seen as a major bottleneck in finding and accessing materials. As I was doing my research, the German national node was running a pilot on a different system called Sample Locator.[5] Two main differences between this platform and the existing Directory concern the data it draws from and the kinds of queries it allows. As interview respondents involved in the development of this system told me, the Locator does not search a central database to which biobanks contribute data, but is directly connected to each biobank itself and thus allows direct searches of what is actually present (or registered as such). It thereby also allows more precise searches. As one person explained to me, in the Directory researchers can search for whether, for example, samples of breast cancer patients and of women of Asian descent are present in any given *biobank*. In the Locator, by contrast, searching for *samples* that meet both criteria—so finding samples from women of Asian descent with breast cancer - would be possible. For this, however, biobanks need to have a standardized local database. The differences between the Directory and the Sample Locator under construction thus bring into focus how research needs, organizational questions (especially regarding centralization and local autonomy) and the technical specifications of biobanking systems intersect in BBMRI-ERIC IT platforms.

In addition to providing IT platforms for finding and accessing stored materials, BBMRI-ERIC is also concerned with the quality of these materials. As several interview respondents indicated, sample quality is important, but not self-evident. Former Director-General Jan-Eric Litton, for example, argued that researchers are often "extremely sloppy" in sample registration, failing to keep information about sample collection, processing and storage. He claims one needs information about "a lot of parameters around the samples and the patients [they came from]". Similarly, a current BBMRI-ERIC staff member argued that researchers often neglect quality management, even though "quality management actually should be the basis". As this person explained, "in principle [we] all have the same aim", which is "to generate, to process, to analyse, to store a sample—and if it is stored, the sample can be re-used. But for that, you have to know everything that happened to the sample prior". Knowing a sample's history and quality is thus a prerequisite for sharing, and since sharing of samples is perhaps the main aim of BBMRI-ERIC, one of the infrastructure's "key elements" is "to provide top-level expertise, services and tools in the area of biobanking" via quality management services (BBMRI-ERIC, 2014, p. 18), This involves quality assessments and the promotion of biobanks "who are able and willing to give access to high quality samples/data" as "an added value and service for both biobanks and their users" (BBMRI-ERIC, 2016d, p. 20).

One important tool BBMRI-ERIC uses for quality assessment is the so-called Self-Assessment Survey (SAS), which "supports biobankers in their efforts to 1) improve sample handling processes 2) implement quality requirements and 3) assess their performance" (BBMRI-ERIC, 2017a, p. 18). An issue of the short-lived *Biobank Europe Magazine* explains the benefits for biobanks of exposing themselves to such an assessment, explaining that the results are remotely monitored by BBMRI-ERIC headquarters and, if positive, marked in the Directory (BBMRI-ERIC, 2017b). According to the 2019 Annual Report, for example, more than sixty surveys had been requested (presumably in 2019, although the report does not specifically mention the timeframe), resulting in 32 quality marks in the Directory (BBMRI-ERIC, 2020, p. 8). According to one staff member, remote auditing requires knowing which questions to ask to find out if biobanks have indeed taken quality management measures, which consist of the implementation of a set of biobanking standards.

Standards are thus vital components of biobanking quality. A "Vision Paper" for BBMRI-ERIC published in 2018 describes quality services as "crucial for the development of personalized medicine solutions, medical devices and diagnostics" (BBMRI-ERIC, 2018), but people working for or with the infrastructure argue that standards are above all important for mundane aspects of research practice. Differences between biobanks in how they handle samples, for example, may create difficulties in collaborations between different biobanks. Growing collaboration across labs and institutions requires samples to be comparable—even as there are significant organizational differences with regard to, for example, whether biobanks are integrated in hospitals or not. But not only samples as such require standardization—so do various other aspects of biobanks including, for example, the samples themselves, sample workflows, etc.

Two brief examples illustrate the kinds of aspects of biobanking standardization may be concerned with. One issue of the *Biobank Europe Magazine* presents the SPIDIA project, which formed an attempt to standardize pre-analytical sample workflows (i.e., how samples are handled before being used in research projects).[6] According to the magazine article, "[t]hese are needed for 1) reducing the number of sample-based diagnostic mistakes, 2) reducing the number of non-reproducible pre-clinical and clinical studies, thus enabling 3) improvement and speeding up of biomarker discoveries and validations" (BBMRI-ERIC, 2017b, pp. 12–13). This example shows how standardizing particular segments of the biobanking process is supposed to help avoid certain high-profile issues in research (i.e., reproducibility—(see, e.g., Baker, 2016)) and contribute to enhancing its productivity (i.e., biomarker discovery).

In our interview, Jan-Eric Litton mentioned a different kind of standard, which he claimed to have helped develop for the Nordic countries, before dispersing it further in Europe. This is the MIABIS standard (see also Tamminen, 2015), which forms a kind of thesaurus that defines key biobanking terms in order to make sure that people refer to the same things when talking about biobanking. This standard has arguably been important for establishing the Europe-wide Directory.

Yet standards specifically are more than an effort to integrate European biobanks, the key aim of BBMRI-ERIC. Rather, so multiple people explained to me, developing standards for Europe alone does not make much sense. One former staff member, for example, stated how "it is clear that Europe cannot develop its own standards, its own little nest. It has to be harmonized with global activities". Science is global, so the tenor of these comments, so standards need to be global, too. More specifically, the development of biobanking standards is a task for the International Standardization Organization (ISO), although BBMRI-ERIC representatives participate in ISO working groups. As one of the infrastructure's Annual Reports legitimates participation in the process of drafting global standards, it "allows BBMRI-ERIC to fulfill its mandate as an international organization in the interest of the European Biobanks" (BBMRI-ERIC, 2016a, p. 4). Efforts at harmonizing medical science in Europe can thus happen via a global detour, too.

Various social science scholars have studied standardization as a technology for shaping social realities, both by producing prescriptions for how to do things and by creating equivalences across time and space (Busch, 2011; Timmermans & Epstein, 2010). In the context of biomedical data or 'bioinformation' in particular, the ability of data and materials to travel is imagined to be an important quality of such data and materials (Metzler et al., 2023), one that depends strongly on standardization (Parry & Greenhough, 2018). Standards are—in principle—voluntary forms of "soft law" that can, in practice, become effectively obligatory (Brunsson & Jacobsson, 2002). Nevertheless, this does not mean that practical implementation of standards is uniform. Standards are often locally contingent, contributing to a changed but not necessarily uniform world (Timmermans & Epstein, 2010). Particularly in the context of European rules and directives, a certain degree of flexibility and subsidiarity often means that "the same" standard or regulation looks different across EU member states (Versluis, 2007). This may also apply to biobanking standards.

Considering the contingency of standardization, it is worth considering what biobanking standards do not do. Although biobanks need to meet certain standards to be able to fully participate in BBMRI-ERIC (e.g., by supplying data according to MIABIS-prescriptions to be added to the Directory), quality criteria as such are not a prerequisite for being able to join. Furthermore, "a standard is not a workflow". This is what a BBMRI-ERIC staff member told me, before explain that

> a standard is not fit-for-all, because some have [sample] transport, some do not have transport [...] you cannot do the same for everyone. But that's what the standard prescribes and then you write your own working process and secure that it meets the standard's requirements.

This person's description of the implementation process illustrates how differences can persist despite standardization. At the same time, one biobank manager explained how standards may also be required based on external factors. This person referred to the introduction of a European regulation for in-vitro diagnostics requiring that testing of such diagnostics would make use of quality-certified samples. This, he argued, turned application of quality standards into a necessity.

This example once more points to the complex intersections between organization and practice in medical research. In a broader sense, BBMRI-ERIC's efforts to create practical change in European biobanking via technologies for making samples visible, accessible and securing their quality involves a continuous balancing act around different views of what biobanking in Europe can and should be, and who can decide, for instance, whether and how samples get shared. While the aim of IT platforms and quality management is the harmonization of sample and data collection(s) for medical research in Europe, the complex and contested nature of these interventions leaves some questions unanswered. What does it mean for research to be 'European'? Which aims should such 'European science' fulfil? And for whose benefit? I turn to these questions next by exploring different answers to the question if and how BBMRI-ERIC works for European research.

(How) Does European Medical Research 'Work'?

A key motivation for establishing BBMRI in the context of the EU's ESFRI research infrastructure promotion policies was to adjust medical science in Europe to the requirements of (post)genomic research, supposedly happening at a larger scale than had previously been the case (Davies et al., 2013). Against this background, the Business Plan that concluded the initial development of the infrastructure argued that

> a key task and challenge for BBMRI-ERIC is to provide access to biological samples and data that properly represent the diversity of European populations and diseases. This can only be achieved by a distributed research infrastructure with operational units in most, if not all, European Member States. (Zatloukal et al., 2012, p. 37)

Here, the aims of BBMRI-ERIC are described in terms of facilitating scientific collaboration in the interest of European population health. To achieve these ends, a distributed research infrastructure is described as the required means. These means are further specified in the various services the infrastructure offers to the European biobanking community—and BBMRI-ERIC regularly argues for its supposed success by providing user numbers for its Directory, Negotiator, quality management and ELSI services.[7] Nevertheless, neither the European character of the infrastructure, nor its contributions to medical research are uncontested.

We have already seen how the European character of BBMRI-ERIC does not mean uniformity across all member states. There are significant differences between countries in biobanking experience and the degree of organization, resulting in divergences in the contributions members make to and expect from the infrastructure. Yet the envisioned membership of most, if not all, EU member states (and beyond, since ERIC membership is not restricted to the EU) has not fully materialized. A number of countries have not, or only recently joined. Two remarkable examples are Luxemburg and Denmark (which have recently joined as an observer), which both have high profile biobanks.[8] As another example, a BBMRI-ERIC staff member in an interview in 2019 referred to Spain, describing it as a "stupid situation, they had one of the most advanced and organized networks of biobanks in Spain, it's super good, but Spain doesn't want to pay for [membership]". This person added that this was mainly due to one person in the responsible ministry, who had just retired. Consequently, Spain joined as an observer soon after. Yet countries do not only decide not to join—two high profile members have left the infrastructure in recent years in the UK (in 2023) and France (in 2020).

Although it is not always entirely clear why countries decide to join or leave BBMRI-ERIC, one staff member indicated in an interview how negotiations with responsible ministries form an important part of the work the headquarter does. As he explained with reference to the ERIC-framework in general, "in the end, it boils down to the interest of the countries". In this person's view, and reflecting the quintessential tension between national and collective interests in European collaboration, this raises questions about how "European" ERIC truly is. As he explained,

ERIC "is still driven by national interests. It looks very European, but [...] it boils down to which country is interested in what". Countries (in this case meaning primarily ministries responsible for science policy) that do not see the value of biobanking, or prioritize other fields of research may thus decide not to spend the BBMRI-ERIC membership fee. For BBMRI-ERIC, this means it needs to make clear why biobanking is an important area for research.

Part of the challenge is to make clear to medical researchers that biobanks—and, in Europe, many of them—exist in the first place and are available as a resource for researchers. One BBMRI-ERIC staff member, for example, explained to me how many large biobanks are well-known, but that this is not the case for many smaller, hospital- or university-based banks that nevertheless have potentially interesting collections. Another person illustrated this problem by explaining how they matched hospitals participating in bone-disease and cancer research to a list of biobanks, finding how researchers "literally don't know that [...] their rare disease ward is on the fourth floor and minus two there is the biobank". The implication is that useful materials and data are unknown and unused, a situation BBMRI-ERIC tries to address by promoting biobanks and making their contents visible and findable. Yet the infrastructure also tries to argue for the importance of biobanking with policy-makers—at both national and European levels. In this regard a staff member explained how

> the [European] Commission is not a thick brick. The research part knows us well, so [we try to] influence the way they, you know, Horizon Europe, the next calls, funding—that kind of stuff and another part is to get BBMRI known [...] to the other parts of the Commission, for example Santé, the health part, they're mostly focused on public health.

Here, BBMRI-ERIC tries to contribute to the visibility of biobanks by making clear how sample and data collections for research ultimately also contribute to public health.

Yet in light of BBMRI-ERIC's hub-and-spoke structure and the aforementioned central role of member states in the governance of ERICs, the relation between the central executive office and the member states is not always unproblematic. Some people I interviewed—particularly representatives of National Nodes—would argue that BBMRI-ERIC is focused too much on European coordination and lobbying, losing sight of the work done in individual biobanks. In this regard, so preparatory phase director Eero Vuorio pointed out to me, member states "who have been funding the collection of samples for tens of years, they have spent tens, maybe hundreds of times more money on the biobanks, their own national biobanks, than they ever pay for BBMRI-ERIC". However, he thereby not only emphasized the importance of the National Nodes, which is something BBMRI-ERIC also does by highlighting national activities in its Annual Reports. Wrapped into his comment is a critique of member states' unwillingness to raise the infrastructure's overall budget. A staff member further explained how the Assembly of Members, in which the member states who pay for the infrastructure make collective decisions, is reluctant to raise membership fees to give the infrastructure more financial leeway. At the same time, so various respondents argued, the current budget is not sufficient to cover the costs of all of BBMRI-ERIC's activities in service delivery, which thus require additional funding from (time-constrained) research project.

These tensions within BBMRI-ERIC member states with regard to what they should fund and why reflects broader uncertainty about what exactly the purpose of a research infrastructure is, particularly with regard to its operational role in research (if any). Bringing this issue to a point, the 2020 Work Programme refers to "a very active debate within the community on the role that research should take within Research Infrastructures" (BBMRI-ERIC, 2019b). It describes research as the "backbone" of biobanking, while simultaneously stating that "the main objective of the funders [i.e., member state governments] is to develop services" (BBMRI-ERIC, 2019b). Should an infrastructure like BBMRI-ERIC be an active participant in research consortia applying for (European) project funding, or should it be an external service provider for successful applicants? According to one staff member, this is also a question related to the aims of European science and research infrastructure policies in general. This person maintained how "at a certain point, there was a plan for these infrastructures to be the pillars, those who implement the European Research Area, the European single market for research". Yet in practice, "something got lost in the middle" and "particularly the ERICs are research organizations coated in something else [...] or grant offices, and that's not sustainable". This person was not convinced that research infrastructures should actively do research and rather sees them in a supporting role.

Based on this distinction between active participation in research and providing support, the question of the significance of research is tied into questions to the particular benefits pursued through BBMRI-ERIC's activities. Respondents also tied these questions into the different background and styles of the first two Directors-General of the infrastructure, Jan-Eric Litton and Erik Steinfelder. While the former came from an academic research background with long-standing involvement in the institutionalization of biobanking in, first, Scandinavia and later Europe more broadly, the latter had an industry background.[9] In interviews, I heard different opinions about whether the transition was a good or a bad thing. Nevertheless, all interview respondents seemed to agree that the shift had had substantial consequences for BMRI-ERIC's strategy. From a primarily research-oriented organization it was said to have become more service-oriented and more tailored towards the potential of biobanks to contribute to the pharmaceutical and biotechnology industries of Europe.

Regardless of how much of this shift can be attributed to the different personalities leading the infrastructure, it seems clear that a strategic reorientation took place at some point. During the first few years of its existence, BBMRI-ERIC promoted itself, for example in an issue of the *Biobank Europe Magazine*, as "a world leading Research Infrastructure for biomedical research in Europe—a true gateway for health" (BBMRI-ERIC, 2017b, p. 18). This notion of a gateway for health was widely used, for example also as a slogan for the *Europe Biobank Week*, a conference jointly organized by BBMRI-ERIC and the international biobanking association ISBER. Yet, a Vision Paper published in 2018 introduced a new lead message, arguing that "BBMRI-ERIC's vision is to further build and strengthen value-added sustainable biobanking for all stakeholders enabling academia and industry to make new treatments possible" (BBMRI-ERIC, 2018). Ever since, BBMRI-ERIC has emphasized "making new treatments possible" as its main message in, for example, its annual reports, work programmes and on its website. While one should be careful with reading too much into what are in essence publicity phrases, the shift from health and research to added value and treatments seems to align with other observations about how—depending on who you ask—the infrastructure changed or "matured". The controversy over these changes, then, is also about what medical research within a research infrastructure entails.

In light of this controversy over the purposes of BBMRI-ERIC and the meaning of research in this context, one person who has been involved with the development of BBMRI-ERIC from early on turned to a specific issue to evaluate its performance. Recalling that a key aim and challenge in establishing the infrastructure had been to facilitate access to samples and data (see, e.g., Litton, 2018), he claimed to see "only minimal improvements". In part, so his belief, this was due to the fact that the infrastructure as such does not own any materials. Furthermore, he saw a "governance problem" in the multiple layers of ERIC, member states, institutions within the member states and, ultimately "groups and institutes that actually have samples and data". To evaluate the impact of this construction, one would thus have to ask "how many samples were collected and how many went into research?" Based on those numbers, "I don't know if it justifies the investments and the efforts, because it doesn't look so great. And one can ask, would it not function quite like that without an infrastructure?" Instead, this person does see value in the coordination, lobbying and research policy activities BBMRI-ERIC has developed.

The modest achievements in sample and data exchange (which are difficult to verify since, as mentioned, BBMRI-ERIC does provide statistics on service use, but not on sample sharing) are linked to issues with sample use and ownership similar to what I encountered in Singapore (see Chap. 3). Jan-Eric Litton describes this issue as "the hugging problem [...] people really like to hug their samples and they [find it] very difficult to share" (see also Tupasela, 2021). Eero Vuorio explained this phenomenon by referring to the time and efforts researchers need to invest in getting funding for a research project and collecting samples, so "it becomes *their* project. And the samples all of a sudden become their samples". From this he concluded how "it is really difficult to find a correct balance between who actually is the owner of the samples and the data. And what kinds of rules one should have to access the data". Here the specific dynamics of how samples and data become valuable for researchers discussed in Chap. 3 (see also Aarden, 2024) run up against the particular contours of how Europe gets made in EU research infrastructure building (Aarden, 2023). The contestation of the centralization of pretty much anything in the European context may mean that in effect not much has changed for how access to materials is granted.

Yet many arguments for the necessity of harmonizing and interconnecting biobanks in Europe do not stop at making access easier. The benefits of a European biobanking infrastructure are ultimately seen in better health and better health care for Europeans. As Jan-Eric Litton summarized the point, "it is extremely important to understand […] we don't do it for making a paper in *Nature*, we do it basically for the patients in Europe". This idea that BBMRI-ERIC ultimately serves European population health can be found in abundance in all kinds of official publications. Yet it raises the question what this European population served by BBMRI-ERIC's efforts is. As contested as the notion of European identity is historically (Delanty, 2002), so difficult it is to draw clear population boundaries in contemporary biomedical research—especially in terms of determining a population for whose benefit research is supposedly done, as Jenny Reardon (2017) has, for example, shown in the context of genomic research in Scotland.

Yet even though there is widespread agreement that strict boundaries between populations do not make much biological sense, long-standing social and cultural imaginations and assumptions about, for instance, Europeans continue to surface in research (Lipphardt, 2010; Bluche et al., 2009; Stuhl et al., 2009). Populations continue to be constructed in biological terms, even though sociopolitical considerations often appear to shape how biological boundaries get drawn (Tupasela, 2017b; Tupasela et al., 2015). This also appears to be the case with references to European population in the context of BBMRI-ERIC. This population is never defined and can perhaps best be understood as the sum of the populations of the infrastructure's (never permanent) set of member states. A European population then serves to legitimate both the construction of a

European biobanking infrastructure (for population health) and the competitive advantages of Europe in this regard (where populations are already sampled and stored through existing public health systems). Specific benefits for this population, however, largely remain clouded by promises and challenges of how to operate an infrastructure for the purpose of medical population research across various layers of operation and organization.

Conclusion: The Institutional and Practical Complexity of European Research

Still doing research during the COVID-19 pandemic, I attended the *Europe Biobank Week* in 2020, which also took place online. One of the event's keynote speakers was the president of the international biobanking organization ISBER. In his talk, he proposed to not think of biobanks as a noun, but *biobanking* as a verb going forward. This intervention suggested that biobanking is about much more than just the collections of samples and data, but also about what researchers (can) do with these materials and about the kinds of capacities and expertise biobankers offers when it comes to the procurement, maintenance and use of biological resources for medical research. Biobankers, he argued, should be careful that biobanks do not turn into "biohoards"—introducing a term that resonates with the aforementioned idea of "sample hugging". In his view, the aim of a biobank should be to release materials for research, which means that a good bank is an empty bank. These claims, made at the most important professional meeting co-organized by BBMRI-ERIC, is but one (albeit significant) manifestation of the idea that biobanks should serve as "sharing nodes" in the international research landscape (Argudo-Portal & Domènech, 2020). The main contribution of biobanks to medical research is thus supposed to lie in sharing, rather than just collecting and storing materials and data.

In this chapter, I explored what medical research comes to be in the context of increasingly strong expectations towards sharing and collaboration, particularly as materialized in the context of EU research infrastructure policies and initiatives. To do so, I analysed three different aspects of the infrastructuring of European biobanking. First, I traced how collaboration and harmonization of medical research in Europe were pursued through the building of a biobanking infrastructure. Next, I looked at how the infrastructure was operationalized through efforts at standardizing sample and data quality and access. Finally, I turned to the question how different actors evaluated the success of BBMRI-ERIC in relation to divergent interpretations of what European science is and is supposed to be. Throughout this discussion, I have highlighted the interpretive flexibility (Bijker & Pinch, 1987) of research as a category that can serve a range of purposes—from expectations of economic benefits associated with ideas of an emerging bioeconomy (Pavone & Goven, 2017; Petersen & Krisjansen, 2015), to expected improvements in public health and healthcare, to science as a means of European integration (Trischler & Kohlrausch, 2014). At the same time, however, what it means to be Europe and the particular dynamics of European collaboration simultaneously shaped how infrastructures incorporating these various purposes could be constructed and operated.

The case of BBMRI-ERIC thus suggests that to ask the question "what is research" means simultaneously asking *where* it is. In other words, looking at both organization and practices of scientific work, which involve much more than just what happens in the lab or at the bench requires considering how these are shaped in and by a particular environment. In the context of European research infrastructures this means not only that infrastructures are built according to specific European rules, but that Europe itself is built simultaneously (Aarden, 2025). BBMRI-ERIC's biography is shaped and directed in critical instances by key moments in EU research infrastructure policy. These policy influences range from the establishment of ESFRI and the publication of its first Roadmap in 2006 and the introduction of the ERIC legal framework in 2009 to financial resources that supported infrastructuring work in the form of funding for the preparatory phase, LPC and ADOPT (as well as numerous other) projects.[10]

Yet, in the ways these policies set the contours for research infrastructures such as BBMRI-ERIC, they simultaneously (re)produced particular ideas of what Europe is. Even in the research context and in spite of the much-repeated argument that research is international, borders continued to matter. Paradoxically, frictions between different jurisdictions or cultures were often cited as a key motivation for building a European biobanking infrastructure, yet nation states remained a main organizational unit in the form of member states. Indeed, national differences continue to be cited as central challenges for and characteristics of European biobanking. Europe, so it seems, continues to be defined by its constituent (national) parts in relation to an elusive communal identity that seems to exist mainly by virtue of shepherding transnational disagreements.

Persistent cross-national differences in Europe further intersect with widespread concerns about sharing materials in biomedical research. Reluctance to share materials is often attributed to individual biobanks or researchers rather than to national differences, leaving some people uncertain about what, exactly, BBMRI-ERIC can contribute to harmonization and collaboration in European biobanking. Such perspectives both suggest that the aim should be to facilitate research through material exchange and raise questions about how a European infrastructure contributes to medical research otherwise. Such debates thereby show what medical research is considered to be, and which role infrastructures for collecting samples and data should have therein. Is research fundamentally an economic activity that should facilitate innovation and competitiveness (i.e., in the form of new treatments)? Should research infrastructures provide basic resources and services to researchers or are they themselves actively involved in doing science? In the context of BBMRI-ERIC, these questions do not appear to have received a definitive answer, keeping the meaning of medical research contested.

Extending this line of thinking, one may also ask who stands to benefit from the making of a European biobanking infrastructure. Within the context of BBMRI-ERIC we find occasional reference to health (care) and to a European population. To some extent, this European population (to be understood, again, as an aggregate of national populations) is the source of Europe's alleged strengths in biobanking. Europe already has sizable sample and data collections available because many countries are said to have long collected materials in the context of national public health programmes and health care arrangements. Yet member states of BBMRI-ERIC differ substantially in terms of what has historically been collected and stored. The narrative of unexplored sample and data goldmines is thus primarily told with reference to the Nordic countries (Tupasela et al., 2020; Cool, 2016). What makes this population European is less evident, nor is it clear how exactly BBMRI-ERIC benefits a European population of any kind. Again, the implicit assumption appears to be a kind of 'trickle down' economics in which investments in medical research will automatically generate new forms of diagnosis and treatment available (and applicable) to 'all'. But similarly to the cases in the previous chapters, there is no immediate consideration of the much more complex and often incomplete pathways via which medical knowledge and innovation may (not) diffuse. To understand how infrastructures for the purpose of medical population research may or may not generate public goods, we thus need to consider what rights and responsibilities for different kinds of people these infrastructures account for.

At one point during our interview, former BBMRI-ERIC DG Jan-Eric Litton explained how the governance structure of BBMRI-ERIC, which tries to balance the interests and concerns of countries big and small, came about. While telling this story, he exclaimed, "I mean, it's Europe. It's extremely complicated". He was referring to the intricacies of the multiple levels of European integration, yet the history and current operations of BBMRI-ERIC show how it is not necessarily more straightforward what 'medical research' is in this context. Similar to Gieryn's (1995, 1999) argument on how the boundaries of science are drawn in situationally specific ways, what medical research means depends on who is making the argument and to what end. Medical research can be multiple things, even at the same time. In the particular context of European research infrastructures, it can furthermore not be separated from its function as a vehicle of European integration. This means that the question what medical research is, is as much of social and political significance as it is relevant to the production of knowledge.

Notes

1. See https://www.esfri.eu/esfri-events/european-research-infrastructures-smarter-future-conference?qt-event=1#qt-event (last accessed 9 July 2025) for details, including videos of sessions. The description here is based on observations made during the event.
2. Referring to the clinical research infrastructure ECRIN and the biobanking infrastructure BBMRI-ERIC—which is the case discussed in this chapter—in particular. These three infrastructures, which Andreu described as "sister organizations" have gradually developed closer collaborations since their establishment over the past two decades.
3. Here referring to BBMRI-ERIC rather than EU member states. We will return to the significance of member states in BBMRI-ERIC below.
4. The host country is where the infrastructure's central administration is located. This country pays an extra fee for this and the infrastructure is in some respects subjects to national legislation. Some of my respondents indicated that having Austria as a host country was less than ideal for this reason, but the country was chosen due to the particular role of Austrian partners in establishing BBMRI.
5. At the time of writing, the Locator exists as one of several sample and data access tools, in addition to the Directory and Negotiator. See https://www.bbmri-eric.eu/bbmri-sample-and-data-portal/ (last accessed 9 July 2025).
6. See also https://www.spidia.eu/ (last accessed 9 July 2025).
7. The 2018 Annual Report (BBMRI-ERIC, 2019a), for example, states that 578 biobanks in 17 countries containing more than 100 million samples contribute to the Directory, which attracts 443 users per month on average. The Negotiator includes 94 biobanks and is on average used 145 times a month, while 88 Self Assessment Surveys were conducted that year, resulting in an additional 15 quality markers. The ELSI Helpdesk, finally, has been able to answer 94.3% of queries it received and has conducted 11 "Ethics Checks" for project applications under the EU Horizon 2020 funding scheme.
8. One interview respondent mentioned IBBL in Luxemburg and Statens Serum in Denmark, along with UK Biobank, explicitly as well-known European biobanks, contrasting them with lesser known biobanks that BBMRI-ERIC could help gain visibility.

9. Jan-Eric Litton was DG from 2013 until 2017 and was succeeded by Erik Steinfelder. Erik Steinfelder returned to an industry position in 2019, before the end of his tenure. After an interim period he was eventually succeeded by Jens Haberman who again came from a more academic-scientific background.
10. For an overview of EU-funded research projects BBMRI-ERIC is involved in, see https://www.bbmri-eric.eu/eu-grants/ (last accessed 9 July 2025).

6

Comparing Infrastructures for the Purpose of Population-Based Medical Research

The case studies in the previous four chapters each focused on a different aspect of what I proposed to call infrastructures for the purpose of population-based medical research. Through this somewhat fragmented approach, I developed this heuristic framework in depth, seeing how such an analysis contributes to further insight into questions of rights, responsibilities and justice in the context of the emergence of promises surrounding practices and governance of 'big' medical research in the early twenty-first century. I therefore analysed case studies in distinct global regions—Asia, Europe and North America—with a focus on different yet prominent domains of medical research, including genomics, the epidemiology of non-communicable diseases and global health. Central to my case studies was the idea of studying *infrastructuring*, which implies not to take institutions and materialities of infrastructure for granted, but to trace how they were built, on the basis of which value commitments and with which epistemic and social effects (Star & Ruhleder, 1996; Karasti & Blomberg, 2018). This means that I focused both on how and why infrastructures were established, organized and funded, on how collection, storage and use of research materials were shaped, and with what expectations towards and outcomes for research participants.

E. Aarden, *Producing Citizenship in Medical Research Collections*, Health, Technology and Society, https://doi.org/10.1007/978-981-95-1707-7_6

In this chapter, I further develop this heuristic conceptually and methodologically. I draw the four case studies together with two aims. First, I explore how the conceptual notions of infrastructure, purpose, population and medical research can illuminate the various case studies. Second, I also attend to the reverse question if and how variation between the cases might contribute to further conceptual development. These two exercises contribute to the conceptual robustness of the analytical perspective, which I believe may be useful for studying further cases of contemporary 'big' medical research across geographical and disciplinary domains. I therefore highlight how this heuristic can be of use in understanding the multiple, sociomaterial, imaginative and situated character of medical research infrastructures. Additionally, I will draw some common threads from my analysis to argue that these cases also provide a particular diagnosis of (public) medical research initiatives at the present time.

My focus on commonalities between the cases in the first part of the chapter invites the opposing question of how to account for differences. I consider this question by discussing some methodological implications of my analysis, focusing on comparison especially. While I see established approaches of cross-national comparison in STS that focus on 'cultures' of and around science and technology as severely limited for my cases (Jasanoff, 2005; Felt et al., 2010), I think comparison can still be a fruitful approach. More particularly, I draw on recent approaches to comparison that suggest that comparing is itself an act of intervention and thus of laying bare or juxtaposing (Fischer, 2018) particular aspects of whichever analytical objects get drawn together to be kept apart (Niewöhner & Scheffer, 2010; Deville et al., 2016). In making these methodological observations, I also point forward to the concluding chapter in which I address the different infrastructures' normative commitments in terms of citizenship.

Analysing Infrastructures for the Purpose of Population-based Medical Research

In the preceding chapters, I have elaborated on the various elements of the analytical heuristic I propose by bringing the analysis of one case of medical tissue and/or data collection in conversation with relevant strands of literature. This approach was partially inspired by Timothy Mitchell's approach in his work on economic expertise in the modernization of Egypt. Mitchell (2002, p. 8) presents his book as a work of political theory where "the theory lies in the complexity of the cases". I do not pretend my analysis to be equally sophisticated, yet think that relevant aspects of the theory may be foregrounded through the cases (which is why I refer to it as heuristic rather than theory throughout). Keeping this in mind, I return to the cases in this section to further excavate aspects of my analysis that might inform work on different cases.

Infrastructures...

The notion of infrastructure served to describe the sociotechnical configuration of research collections. These configurations included two complementary aspects that have been widely discussed in the literature in infrastructure studies (Slota & Bowker, 2017; Anand et al., 2018). These include, on the one hand, infrastructures as background work that allow continued research and the circulation of data and tissue, and the imaginative properties of infrastructure on the other, which frame it as a vehicle of promise and progress.

The infrastructure concept framed my discussion of the Framingham Heart Study, which was established in the late 1940s in the United States to study causes and contributing factors of cardiovascular disease. The beginnings of the study were largely experimental, requiring several years of finding out both which institutions would be involved and what the appropriate study method would be (Oppenheimer, 2005). However, from the very beginning the study was imagined as a long-term resource for studying cardiovascular disease and was indeed continued beyond its initial 20-year timeframe—albeit on the basis of some organizational reforms and the inclusion of new approaches (Patel, 2012). Nevertheless, key aspects of the study infrastructure have remained largely stable. These include the emphasis on randomly selected participants and the prospective study of disease, its focus on individual risk factors and its lack of ethnic diversity. These aspects persist even at present where, although various research and administrators signal a shift towards increased emphasis on genetic factors, these are still largely framed within the established approach of lifestyle-based predispositions.

At the same time, the Framingham Heart Study provides insight into the imaginative dimensions of medical research infrastructures. On the one hand, the study is widely publicized as, and considered to be, a landmark in the investigation not only of cardiovascular disease, but of chronic disease epidemiology more broadly (Roberts, 2000). This status of the study has ramifications for its present operations, since its materials and data are highly desired by researchers elsewhere. The study's particular status, then, can for example be deduced from the early inclusion of all of its core data in the dbGaP research database. But exchange and reuse of data in other studies is also restricted by another highly valued, symbolic dimension of the study as infrastructure, which is its tie-in with the local community. The contributions of Framingham residents and their families (particularly in two subsequent generation cohorts) are regularly highlighted in the context of the study and seen as both an advantage (e.g., for genetic research) and, occasionally, disadvantage (e.g., for doing research on socioeconomic factors). Interestingly, the symbolic significance of the study's community base has taken on renewed significance in relation to genetic research and a recognition (at least as narrated by people involved with the study) of the value of families in comparison to large, but unrelated population samples.

The designation 'infrastructure' is only formalized (twice over!) in the European biobanking infrastructure BBMRI-ERIC, although this does not necessarily mean the meaning of infrastructure is any clearer. It is rather contested in terms of how the idea of an infrastructure gets realized. On the one hand, the functionality of the infrastructure is questioned in terms of its limited contribution (in some eyes) to the circulation of samples or in supporting rather than doing research. On the other hand, the infrastructure is highly symbolic as a manifestation of European research policy, even though its European character is questioned on the basis of the complex, multi-layered 'hub-and-spoke' structure in which European agendas do not always align with those of member states or individual biobanks.

The infrastructure of the Million Death Study is somewhat paradoxical, as the study embodies both a critique of India's public health and civil registration infrastructures, while simultaneously relying on a demographic infrastructure (the SRS) for data collection. But the study involves various other elements for building a functional knowledge production infrastructure under conditions with limited resources. Material elements such as software platforms and discursive elements like the various instructions for accurate data collection or diagnosis jointly make the production of medical knowledge that does not rely on the health system, nor on advanced research techniques, possible. At the same time, this infrastructure incorporates various promises with regard to addressing pressing health problems for India and the global South. As a relatively low cost method (at its most extreme described as a "simple conversation") verbal autopsy contains the promise of enabling the generation of accurate mortality statistics in low resource settings. This promise also entails the idea of informing the formulation of better health policy, although there is some ambivalence in how this relates to diagnostic shortcomings a method relying on narrated symptoms may have (Aarden, 2019).

Finally, the Singapore Tissue Network might be characterized as an infrastructure that remained experimental (Bruun Jensen & Morita, 2015), never quite succeeding in establishing background routines for the circulation or sharing of samples. The design of the network nevertheless entailed quite specific ideas of how the circulation of materials could be facilitated. These relied primarily on the imagined contribution of a centralized tissue repository to scientific collaboration, itself seen as a precondition for economic productivity. The Singapore Tissue Network therefore prioritized the quality of sample storage and retrieval in an automated facility located at the Biopolis research campus. Most notably, data were not included as they were imagined to form the groundwork for collaboration if obtained directly from a potential research partner. Yet the particular imaginary of collaboration inscribed in the network did not align with how researchers believed a repository ought to function. They accepted the economic aims of biomedical research and a high-quality storage facility, but not the loss of control over their materials. For them, familiarity and trust towards both donors/participants and collaborators were vital characteristics of the functionality of a tissue storage infrastructure.

These various examples of infrastructures thereby show how the analytical separation between function and imagination is difficult to maintain. Each in their own way, these infrastructures tie the materiality of knowledge production (Latour & Woolgar, 1986) to meanings of knowledge (Reardon, 2017). The exact configurations of these tie-ins can be quite different—they do, for example, tie in the state, or state(-like) institutions in distinct ways. In some cases, policy visions of infrastructures conflict with those of scientific practitioners, but we find other lines of conflict as well. Overall, using the notion of infrastructure shows the manifold ways sociomaterial configurations for producing knowledge may both reflect and shape hopes and promises of social progress.

… for the Purpose…

The purposes of tissue and data collection, as well as of medical research writ large, extend beyond the mere accumulation of knowledge in each of these cases. Different forms of value are imagined and pursued in medical research infrastructures. In many cases, views of (future) value are embedded in broader sociotechnical imaginaries (Jasanoff & Kim, 2015) of the ways science and technology contribute to desirable social futures. Such imaginaries exist in interaction with imaginaries of how science works or should work (Marcus, 1995), but also with processes of value generation. The value of a collection is not given in advance, but produced in processes of collecting, storing, using and otherwise working with data and materials (Dussauge et al., 2015b). Moreover, in a research context such value is not necessarily only epistemic or economic, but can take on a variety of—often conflicting—shapes (Pinel et al., 2020).

The Singapore Tissue Network was characterized by a clear orientation towards, primarily economic, value creation. This orientation can in turn be located in the context of an established imaginary of economic growth and social well-being rooted in the development of ever-more technologically advanced sectors of industry and technology development in Singapore (Low, 2004). In the specific context of the Biomedical Sciences Initiative, this imaginary was linked to specific characteristics of the Singapore population as representative of diversity in Asia (Ong, 2013).

Nevertheless, this diversity was not deliberately pursued in the collection of samples for the Singapore Tissue Network. The network contained samples collected in research projects funded by national funding agencies. The aim of the network was to facilitate sharing of and collaboration with the collected materials, for which the design of the repository was supposed to provide incentives.

The particular imaginary underwriting the Singapore Tissue Network and its approach to producing value resulted in the closure of the repository after a decade. This is largely due to the contested view of value generation enacted through the repository. Researchers contributing samples or interested in working with them held different views of how materials would be made valuable. On the one hand, they attached more importance to the specific means by which samples were collected. These would not always enable direct generation of value—for example when collecting tumour tissue that had no immediate application, but might be needed for research at some point in the future. Yet these practitioners also held different views of how materials could be made valuable. Whereas the Singapore Tissue Network was based on the idea that researchers interested in using samples would contact the contributors who possessed relevant data, researchers considered existing familiarity with such colleagues a precondition for collaboration. They thereby attached a range of other values to tissue than just its potential productivity in research, considering, for example, the trustworthiness of the person who collected the tissue, but also their own career interests, how use of materials could enhance the (scientific) value of a collection, and more. These issues were not part of the imagined value production processes designed into the network, resulting in a lack of use that is widely cited as the cause for its termination.

The Framingham Heart Study started with the purpose of identifying characteristics of the individual that contributed to the emergence of cardiovascular disease over time. From the very beginning, study hypotheses were formulated such that individual behaviour was most intensely studied and thereby soon singled out as the main (set of) causes, dubbed risk factors. Over time, the study identified ever more complex factors contributing to cardiovascular disease, for example by tracing different patterns of disease in families. Yet the focus on individual behaviour remained remarkably consistent even in relation to genetic predispositions. As a result, the study has been criticized for its focus on individual risk factors at the expense of other, social determinants of disease (Aronowitz, 1998; Rothstein, 2003)—particularly in light of its narrow racial profile and the inclusion of structural factors in studies of cardiovascular disease in African American communities that are modelled on the Framingham Heart Study (Pollock, 2012).

The purposes of the European biobanking infrastructure BBMRI-ERIC are remarkably similar to those of the STN, yet take on a particular shape. Standardization and harmonization of biobanking practices in the interest of scientific collaboration formed an important motivation for developing this infrastructure, but it does not involve centralization of collections like STN did. Moreover, BBMRI-ERIC builds on a distinct imaginary of European integration in the context of EU research policy. Central to this imaginary and how it pursues integration is the ongoing challenge of balancing communal European interests with the interests of individual member states. However, the idea that this form of European integration can enhance scientific collaboration is contested. Not only do some people raise doubts with regard to the different interests that actors involved with BBMRI-ERIC pursue, but some also argue that the particular way the infrastructure seeks to promote collaboration and sample sharing does not actually work.

The Million Death Study builds in part on a negative imaginary of the shortcomings of the state in mobilizing science for public welfare, but ties this to the idea that the purpose of improved public health may be achieved by using a low-cost method for producing more accurate and representative mortality statistics. This should be achieved by operating a fine-grained infrastructure for data collection and analysis that can ultimately generate cause of death statistics that are good enough to inform policy-making. This approach is contested on the basis of its methodological limitations in producing fully secure diagnoses. Yet for researchers in the study this is of lesser concern. Since they see it as their aim to improve public health and to provide numbers in support that are better than what has thus far been available, they find an approximation of gold standard diagnostics acceptable. Here, the particular purpose of the study is reflected in how data generation through the verbal autopsy method is valued.

In each of these case studies particular scientific, medical or economic purposes are imagined in relation to a broader imaginary of the possible societal benefits science and technology may generate. To turn such imaginaries into realities, particular imaginations of how to do science inform practices of value production—with value taking on various different forms. But in each of the cases, either purposes themselves or the mechanism through which they should be achieved are contested. In many cases, this involves a questioning of whether a particular strategy (say, verbal autopsy in the MDS) can actually deliver on its purpose (to provide better mortality data). Contestations around the purposes of each of these infrastructures thus show how multiple interpretations of the benefits of infrastructuring research are possible.

... of Population-Based...

Population forms a key, if often implicit, reference point for all medical research collections. Population is often defined in a narrow, technical way (Krieger, 2012), even though no population can be included without at least some considerations of how its broader social characteristics feature into recruitment for research (Tupasela et al., 2015). At the same time, sampling a population and collecting research materials in the age of big biology implies that population is turned into data in specific ways. Datafication of a population (Mejias & Couldry, 2019) involves both the questions how to turn individuals into a set of characteristics considered relevant for research and how to classify it as a collective (Bowker & Star, 1999). How populations get framed or made thereby directly affects for whom research is beneficial at both an individual and a collective level.

Reference to a national population that has not previously been adequately captured is at the heart of the Million Death Study. In this study, the population gets defined and redefined in various steps, involving both fragmentation and integration of characteristics that collectively define population. The study forms a response to a perceived lack of accurate cause of death statistics on the Indian population. To correct this issue and provide data that can be considered representative of the population, the study relies on an existing population sample for tracing births, deaths and migration in India. A method called verbal autopsy is applied to collect data on the circumstances surrounding each death in the sample on the basis of a household interview. This symptomatic data is used to allow two physicians to diagnose an individual cause of death, and all individual causes are aggregated to form a national overview of mortality that can be further parsed by region or be considered exemplary for other low- and middle-income countries.

In the process of data generation and processing, population gets de- and reconstructed at various points. First of all, the Indian population in the SRS is supposed to be represented by less than 1% of its total number, although this fraction is selected on the basis of specific criteria. In this sample, a supposedly representative number of deaths is turned into a set of symptomatic descriptions or data points based on responses to structured interview questions. These symptoms occurring around the time of death are pieced together into one cause of death in a coding process that includes steps to arrive at one unique cause. Individual causes of death then are integrated into population-wide mortality statistics. They supposedly describe the population's health status accurately, indicating, for example, which health problems are more or less common than previously believed. This process involves the classification of deaths as unique events into comparable 'causes' as prescribed by the ICD-10 system. Deaths thereby become meaningful for public health policy, as they inform the measures that should be taken. All of the steps in this process further rely on a range of data technologies, which are increasingly imagined at a higher degree of technical sophistication. Not only do software platforms increasingly guide physicians' diagnostic decision-making, the ideal is that at some point machines can entirely take over the role of determining what India's population dies from.

In the Singapore Tissue Network, the specific profile of the population from which samples were collected appeared to be of limited relevance. Although Singapore's ethnic diversity, and the supposed representation of the main Asian population groups in its administrative classification of Chinese, Indians and Malays is used to argue for the country's possible contributions to medical research (Ong, 2015), there was no deliberate recruitment for the STN on any basis. Things look slightly different when looking at the recruitment of populations in individual studies or repositories. Ethnicity plays a role in recruitment for epidemiological studies, even though its relevance in medical terms is unclear (Coopmans & Tan, 2018). But at the very least, ethnicity matters socially in the context of recruitment. However, other aspects of a population matter, too—for example, the kinds of diseases people suffer from are a main decision criteria in deciding whom to take tumour tissue from in 'unscheduled' sample collection. In Singapore, the population thus mainly exists as an abstract entity that may benefit from—but, as social science critiques suggest (Waldby, 2009a; Holden & Demeritt, 2008)—is also expected to contribute to, medical research.

The population sample included in the Framingham Heart Study is also not seen to be representative of the US population as a whole, and some even explicitly deny the relevance of such representativeness. More important to how the population of participants in this study is defined are its characteristics as members of a community and of families. The notion of community forms a backbone of (public) representations of the study in which it is suggested that this particular characteristic of the participating sample has allowed the study to continue for multiple decades. The inclusion of families as defined on the basis of both biological and marital relatedness has gained particular significance in the context of genetic research, where familial patterns of disease may be traced and linked to possible genetic factors. Biologically unrelated spouses in the sample are understood as control groups for such research. At the same time, relevant characteristics of the population are inscribed in the minutiae of epidemiological research methods and findings. Random population sampling and a focus on individual behaviour as causes of disease that may nevertheless take on epidemic collective proportions are stalwarts of the Framingham conception of health and disease—all while, as noticed, marginalizing both biological and social aspects of racial difference.

BBMRI-ERIC does not, as such, have a strategy for including a particular population in its collection, since the infrastructure does not collect or store any samples of its own. As a network of biobanks, there are surely different recruitment strategies among its member biobanks. It matters, for example, whether a biobank is focused on specific diseases or aims to build a general resource for medical research on a given (national) population. Yet, the absence of any explicit population recruitment does not mean that there is no reference to a population with BBMRI-ERIC. In public appearances, the infrastructure not so rarely erects a presumed European population as its supposed point of reference. This European population is, in part, positioned as its audience and beneficiary, as seen in expressions of, for instance, European patients as the collective for whom investments in BBMRI-ERIC are ultimately made. Similarly, albeit more implicitly, the European population also forms the point of reference for legitimating the infrastructure. The availability of samples from this population, collected and stored in the context of health care systems characteristic of the European social fabric, is presented as a clear competitive advantage for Europe. This diffuse idea of a European population thereby does a lot of work in the rhetoric of BBMRI-ERIC, if not in the collection practices of its constituent biobanks in different member states.

Population can thereby take on a number of different shapes in medical research infrastructures, ranging from specific, representative collectives captured in samples or data to rather more evasive rhetorical points of reference. The multiple and elusive forms populations may take thereby suggest that the question who benefits from medical research often does not have a straightforward or specific answer. I will return to this issue in the next chapter; for now, it is worth noting that the less specified the population recruited to participate in research, the more implicit the collective of beneficiaries appears to be as well.

...Medical Research

The question what medical research is generated quite distinct answers in the four case studies. Different research objects and practices of knowledge production reflect different understandings of research. On the one hand, the distinct meanings of medical research are associated with broader transformations in science towards increased consideration of the social and economic uses of knowledge (Guston, 2000; Hessels et al., 2009). On the other hand, the cases show the complex and intricate institutional and practical configuration of research, which is for example reflected in the use of standards delineating particular preferential approaches to the making and evaluation of knowledge claims (Busch, 2011). Various medical research infrastructures consequently incorporate distinct meanings of what research may be. These are not seldomly also in conflict within single infrastructures.

Several fault lines characterize the multiple meanings of medical research within BBMRI-ERIC. As a formally designated infrastructure, BBMRI-ERIC first and foremost defines its particular role in research as distinct from that of more time-constrained and output-driven projects. This in spite of the prominent role of EU-funded research projects in the establishment of BBMRI-ERIC and in its ongoing operations. This, in turn, points to a second fault line that revolves around the role an infrastructure like this should have in medical research. This can be a role either as facilitator or as active participant in research projects, a distinction that also relates to how BBMRI-ERIC's contribution to the European research landscape at large is imagined. Tied into these discussions of how an infrastructure should figure into medical research is a question of what its contribution to research should be at a more substantive level, as characterized by the opposition between a primarily scientific orientation and an orientation towards innovation and marketable products.

These multiple, contested meanings of research within BBMRI-ERIC are also related to the infrastructure's organizational configuration. The multi-layered governance and operations of this infrastructure finds expression in a variety of often conflicting ideas of what it is for. One interview respondent expressed their amazement at the tensions within member states, observing how government representatives in the Assembly of Members were focused on service delivery, whereas scientists in the National Nodes prioritized support in doing research. This organizational complexity was also reflected in the various services for quality management and the visibility and accessibility of samples that BBMRI-ERIC developed. Although BBMRI-ERIC was actively involved in the development of quality standards, these do not in and of themselves result in the harmonization of biobanking practices. Similarly, making materials visible and accessible through the Directory and Negotiator platforms depended on the willingness of individual biobanks to supply the required information on their collections. These are just some examples of the complex shape medical research takes in the context of a European research infrastructure. This is in part a result of the rather broad and ill-defined status of such infrastructures (Cramer et al., 2020) and the limited consideration of the particular issues of concern in specific scientific fields in European regulation (Reichel, 2015).

The Million Death Study is situated at the intersection of different approaches to and meanings of medical research. On the one hand, the study was established in explicit contrast to a specific form of medical research, the collection of mortality statistics within the health system. On the other hand, the study involves the development of a specific novel form of research relying on verbal autopsy data, entangled with an established and growing environment of global health research involving funding from and collaboration with research institutions in the global North (Crane, 2010). Medical research in the Million Death Study is integrated with the demographic data collection techniques of the SRS. Overall, data is central to the study, be it in the form of symptomatic data points or the particular diagnoses that form the basis of aggregate mortality statistics and (supposedly) health policy measures based thereon. This centrality of data is further reflected in the considerable weight given to data quality control in both re-sampling of a subset of VA records and self-assessment of diagnoses by coding physicians. Yet the meaning of research is also contested and refined in relation to the study's purposes where diagnostic accuracy (i.e., a gold standard) is ultimately seen as secondary to the usefulness of study results for public health.

In relation to the Singapore Tissue Network and the BMSI, medical research was quite prominently considered an economic activity. The idea that a main motivation for funding research and establishing research institutions and support structures was to facilitate economic growth does not seem to be very controversial in Singapore. Controversy rather emerged around the question how medical research should be conducted to realize this aim. The design and operations of the Singapore Tissue Network seem to suggest a belief in a rather direct and functional relation between tissue storage and economic growth. This was also evident in how the logic of how STN worked was described in interviews. Samples in the repository were supposed to draw interest, yet to be able to do research with these samples required collaboration with other researchers who held the relevant clinical data. This approach conflicted with the more relational understanding of how research and scientific collaboration worked among scientists. This relational understanding is illustrated by the statement that science needs heroes and the emphasis on negotiations as part of the process of gaining access to materials.

According to various publications celebrating the Framingham Heart Study, finally, this infrastructure made a central contribution to defining what contemporary medical research should be. Its randomized and prospective approach counts as a main methodological innovation in epidemiology (Epstein, 1992), even though the initial sample was not entirely random (and almost exclusively based on people of white European descent). At present, the study's multigenerational cohorts along with the availability of longitudinal datasets are presented as important strengths of the study, particularly in the context of genomic research. Furthermore, it is striking how a study to which many ascribe a historical reputation of unwillingness to share data has become part of complex international networks of knowledge production. At the same time, the robust status of the Framingham Heart Study as the essence of modern epidemiology obscures the many exclusions this study design entails. Aside from its ethnically narrow sample, its specific methodological orientations prioritize measurable individual behavioural characteristics at the expense of the role of more complex, 'social determinants' of health.

Medical research may appear to be a rather straightforward category on the surface, one that describes processes of knowledge-making with regard to risks, causes, progression and cures for disease. Instead, I focused my analysis on the various organizational forms medical research may take and how these (mis)align with particular ideas regarding why such research is done. From this vantage point, medical research can be a number of different things, in some cases within the same infrastructure at the same time, and often valued differently by distinct actors. In relation to the broader understanding of population research infrastructures and their purposes I investigated here, such variety in the meanings of medical research suggests that how research is organized and done is connected to particular situated value commitments engrained in scientific practice.

Conceptualizing Infrastructures for the Purpose of Population-based Medical Research

The discussion in the previous section shows both the diverse and complex meanings of infrastructures for the purpose of population-based medical research and the close intertwinements of the various aspects of these infrastructures in each of them (see Table 6.1). I will therefore use this section to structure my observations along two axes. On the one hand, I draw together some analytical observations about the kinds of phenomena these infrastructures are. On the other hand, I want to take my observations to distil some key characteristics of 'big' medical science at the present time. I will therefore first argue that infrastructures for the purpose of population-based medical research can be understood to be sociomaterial, multiple, imaginative and situated before positioning them in relation to the contemporary state, economy, society and to data.

Infrastructures for the purpose of population-based medical research can be characterized as sociomaterial with reference to the relations between actors, institutions, routines, tools, techniques, methods and so on that jointly shape how research on populations gets done.[1] The social and the material thereby mutually configure one another to create particular forms of research practice and governance. This is, for example, visible in the way the Directory and Negotiator platforms of BBMRI-ERIC incorporate the relations between a central European organization and individual biobanks, or in the way relations with and within a multigenerational local community both shape which materials get collected and stored in the Framingham Heart Study, but also under which conditions these materials become available for outside researchers. The observation of sociomaterial infrastructures thereby suggests that tissue and data collections can never be seen separate from their particular sociopolitical location, but are at the same time not reducible to sociopolitical priorities or interests. The material making of a population and of population health—be it in the form of blood or solid tissue samples, quality assessment criteria, symptomatic questionnaires or other techniques—thus plays a pivotal role in shaping what health means and whose health

Table 6.1 An overview of the analytical heuristic for each case study

	FHS	STN	MDS	BBMRI-ERIC
Infrastructures	Multigenerational repository; community and family-centred research model	Research support structure; contested contribution to economic growth	Application of demographic sample and VA method; low-cost model for global South	Aimed at harmonizing biobanking; formally designated in EU policy
Purpose	Identifying coronary prone individual; contested for narrow framing risk and ethnicity	Facilitating collaboration for economic productivity; contested value-making processes	Producing reliable mortality statistics for better health policy; contested over accuracy	Harmonizing biobanking and integrating science; contested over effectiveness
Population based	As community and families; at-risk individuals	As Asian tissue; ethnic recruitment in research projects	As data; representative demographic sample	As tissue and data; collected in member biobanks
Medical research	Shifting focus on disease mechanisms over time	How productivity and research practice relate	Representative statistics for policy improvement	Balancing aims and European interests

is considered (or not) in medical research. The production of medical knowledge, the governance of science and the politics of medical knowledge thus intersect in both the relations built within and around these infrastructures and their material form.

Secondly, these infrastructures can be described as multiple. Drawing on Annemarie Mol's (2003) work on multiplicity in medical practice this notion refers not just to different meanings they can have, but how single infrastructures can be different things at the same time. These different things are made in practices—of, for example, diagnosing, treating or experiencing the disease atherosclerosis in Mol's study. Here I use the idea of multiplicity to illustrate how frictions may emerge in medical research that are not the result of differences in understanding alone. BBMRI-ERIC is a case in point; the infrastructure may be aimed at developing services and thus be successful in its work of providing quality management, IT and ELSI support for some, whereas it less successfully serves to facilitate sample exchange for others. Similarly, the Million Death Study may only provide imperfect mortality data when focusing on clinically confirmed medical knowledge, while delivering highly important and relevant insights if seen in terms of its contributions to health policy making in India. Understanding medical population research infrastructures as multiple, then, opens up the possibility of analysing how particular configurations may generate different kinds of benefits at the same time, not all of which serve 'the same' publics. Such ontological politics (Mol, 1999) suggest that it depends on the practical doing of research infrastructures if and how they generate a public good.

While the multiplicity of infrastructures points to the politics of practices, their various different dimensions are also entangled with imaginaries—of what infrastructures may produce, what their purposes are, how they serve particular populations and what medical research entails. The imaginative dimension of infrastructures draws on Sheila Jasanoff and Sang-hyun Kim's (2009, 2015) concept of sociotechnical imaginaries that illustrates how scientific and technological projects reflect particular designs for social progress. Within the cases of medical research infrastructures presented here, imaginaries are not only performed by social collectives, but also designed into how the infrastructures work. Moreover, as with the multiplicity of the infrastructures themselves, the various collectives that (more or less explicitly) formulate imaginaries for research infrastructures may be fragmented and imagine things in divergent and often conflicting ways (Kim, 2013). This is obviously the case in the context of the Singapore Tissue Network and its divergent imaginaries of how value could be produced from stored materials. Here, imaginaries of complex practices of value generation in repositories conflicted with the expectation that stored materials were valuable as such. By contrast, the Million Death Study was based on an imaginary of the shortcomings of existing methods for generating mortality statistics. This imaginary of deficiency was confronted by developing an alternative approach to measuring mortality that reinvented the entire process. The Million Death Study can therefore be taken as a reflection of the way imaginaries of and in research infrastructures shape and are shaped by the various different elements of such infrastructures—ranging, in this case, from the sample used, to the methods for data collection and the particular meaning attributed to the study's outcomes. Imaginaries are thereby not merely a matter of collective visions and design, but touch ground in how research within particular infrastructures gets done.

Finally, infrastructures for the purpose of population-based medical research are situated. I will return to the point that this does not mean that they are manifestations of particular national cultures. Rather, the particular form and workings of these infrastructures is shaped by the actors and institutions that shape them. These surely reflect specific institutional and regulatory conditions of the places where they get established—although these conditions are by no means set by national authorities alone—but also the particular priorities of, for example, medical research disciplines. Along these lines, the Framingham Heart Study is rooted in the mid-twentieth century medical research landscape of the (northeastern) United States and the broader emergence of novel epidemiological approaches to chronic disease at the time. It has since developed from that basis, periodically adjusting to both the changing regulatory and funding landscape of medical research as well as the emergence of new approaches in medical research. On the other side of the spectrum of longevity, the Singapore Tissue Network reflects approaches to economic growth typical to Singapore, but also broader trends regarding the economic potential attributed to biobanks around the turn of the century. Moreover, the practices of recruitment and collection themselves were articulated in terms of both ongoing social transformations in Singapore and of Singapore's position in the region (in the form of hiring qualified pathologists from surrounding lower wage countries). Consequently, these infrastructures and the ways they work are significantly shaped by different characteristics of their geographical-political and scientific environments.

The situated nature of these infrastructures further suggests that they should reflect certain characteristics of the contemporary politics of medical research practices. On the basis of my analysis, I would like to emphasize four aspects in particular. The first of these concerns the particular relation of these infrastructures to the state. Although there is much ongoing discussion about the supposed decreasing relevance of the state, all of these infrastructures relate to the state, or state(like) institutions in particular ways. This may likely be an effect of their (largely) public funding, administration and operation. But rather than only demonstrating the continued relevance of the state in the early twenty-first century, each of these cases also contributes to shaping what the state may mean at present. BBMRI-ERIC is part of the major and contested state-making project of the European Union while also clearly showing the continued relevance of the nation states that constitute this overarching entity. The Million Death Study both highlights failures of the state and seeks to reconstruct it through other means. The active role of the state in pursuing economic development was critical to both the establishment and termination of the Singapore Tissue Network, and the complicated relation between the state and health in the United States is in part maintained through the focus on community, family and individual in the Framingham Heart Study.

If the state is considered less relevant in the context of medical research this is in part related to hypotheses of a decline of the welfare state as a locus of much population-based research and the emergence of private industry as an alternative. This hypothesis is in part related to the idea of an emerging bioeconomy, although the bioeconomy is substantially entangled with state investments in research and innovation (Goven & Pavone, 2015). Nevertheless, ongoing social science debates about the role of capital and commodification in the life sciences resonates with the case studies presented here. Part of the debate focuses on the question whether tissue and data form commodities or assets for value creation (Birch & Tyfield, 2013; Chiapetta & Birch, 2018). Although I do not focus explicitly on how economic value gets generated in medical research in my analysis, the cases largely reflect imaginations of wealth to be generated from research. This is most explicitly the case for the Singapore Tissue Network, but also quite prominent in BBMRI-ERIC, particularly in light of its strategic shift towards "making new treatments possible" (BBMRI-ERIC, 2018). That economic profitability can also be a source of controversy became visible in the context of the Framingham Heart Study, where concern about participant dropout provides a reminder of the different kinds of value that may be associated with medical data. Economic value of data or other medical resources was no topic of conversation in the Million Death Study, and yet studies of philanthrocapitalism in global health (such as the Gates Foundation, which is also involved with the MDS) have suggested that contributions to global health serve in part to protect donors' economic interests (McGoey, 2015)—see also Sunder Rajan (2015) on the complex relation between philanthropy and intellectual property in pharmaceutical innovation.

Beyond the speculative economic value of medical tissue and data collections, the cases further suggest some resonance with changing social contracts for science (Gibbons, 1999; Aarden, 2017a). David Guston (2000) originally proposed the notion of a social contract for science to describe a particular period in US science policy after the Second World War in which blanket funding for science was expected to generate unspecified societal benefits. Beyond this use, I find the concept useful to think through various (relatively) recent diagnoses of an increased demand for social relevance, usefulness and responsiveness for scientific research (see, e.g., Hessels & Van Lente, 2008 for an overview). The various cases included here each quite explicitly profess a form of social value, mostly in terms of generating better health, economic progress or (scientific) proficiency and competitiveness. But the related question if and how these infrastructures are subject to some form of public evaluation is less clear cut. The Framingham Heart Study reforms in the early 1970s were explicitly informed by stricter evaluations of NIH spending, and the Singapore Tissue Network, too, was closed—along with some other facilities (Nature, 2010)—once the BMSI was expected to become economically productive. BBMRI-ERIC has integrated such questions into the organization by ways of a Stakeholder Forum, and one could argue that the evaluation of the Million Death Study lies in part in the formulation of health programmes in India. The question of public evaluation of research is one I return to in the concluding chapter.

One final observation here concerns how the cases do or do not reflect the emergence of big data and of 'data-centric' biology (Leonelli, 2016). There are certainly traces of this trend in the context of the two cases that revolve around (genomic) biobanks. The question of data and how to facilitate its findability, accessibility and reuse (Wilkinson et al., 2016) form a major area of work in BBMRI-ERIC. The importance of data is somewhat ironic in the context of the Singapore Tissue Network, where it was the decision not to include data in the biobank itself that accentuated some of the issues eventually resulting in it getting shut down. But the other two cases also provide insight into the significance and, perhaps especially, complexity of 'big data' in medical research at present. Some Framingham researchers would explicitly contrast their study with more obviously big projects such as national biobanks to argue for the value of 'smaller', but more interconnected datasets. Again, this was an argument for the scientific value of families, but also of longitudinal data. Judging by the estimate of over one million blood samples kept from the study, however, one can argue about the size of the dataset even if it comes from a relatively limited number of participants. In the Million Death Study, by contrast, the size of the (desired) dataset is not only part of how the study got its name, but also made very explicit in projections of the study's future. Here I found explicit reference to big data, algorithms and machine learning, all of which seem to reflect a belief that medical research moves towards cheaper and faster processing of symptomatic data points—even though at the time human physicians' pattern recognition was still better than that of machines.

These various perspectives on the size of datasets and its significance raise the question what the 'big' in big biology stands for—total amounts of data, number of participants, complexity of data, or something else still.[2] Rather than answering this question, Kaushik Sunder Rajan (2013, p. 486) has suggested that the label 'big' is "a placeholder and polymorphic signifier" for a more diverse and complex set of transformations in the life sciences, similar to what I have suggested for medical research collections in this section. Identifying such transformations across different cases, but in distinct ways, further raises questions regarding the meaning of 'the global' in medical research and if and how comparison can be a fruitful analytical strategy. I turn to these questions next.

Doing Comparison in 'Global' Science

Each of the cases presented previously suggests that medical research increasingly moves beyond national borders. This appears a straightforward observation on the surface, but it does raise some questions about scale. Border-crossing takes the shape of collaboration between nation-states in BBMRI-ERIC, but also has a more diffuse dimension both there and in the other cases. Both the Million Death Study and the Singapore Tissue Network were positioned in a particular international context. In the latter case, this was about Asia, in terms of both the diverse ethnic profile of its population and its position as a gateway to Asian markets for the pharmaceutical industry. In the former case, it reflects the idea of both biological and socioeconomic diversity in India as a mirror of differences in mortality profiles across the global South. Both cases thereby also have a hint of a 'global' dimension, yet this is brought forward most explicitly in the Framingham Heart Study, which is positioned as a global model for cardiovascular epidemiology (Greenberg, 2010).

The notion of the global, however, is never unproblematic. In a broad sense, 'the global' is never fully independent of 'the local' and both develop together and in relation to other scales to create overlapping spatio-temporal orders (Sassen, 2000) that Stephen Collier and Aihwa Ong (2005) have described as "global assemblages". They thereby refer to how the global takes specific form in particular locations, causing human existence to become "subject to technological, political and ethical reflection and intervention" (Collier & Ong, 2005, p. 4). Reflecting more specifically on the circulation of people and ideas—increasingly including to and from the global South—in the sciences, Michael Fischer (2007, p. 574) posits the idea of "emergent cosmopolitan scientific worlds". These too, Fischer argues, involve "local ecologies, synergies, and networks of knowledge production" that should be analysed to understand if and how science has become increasingly 'global'.

The cross-border circulation of scientific ideas, people, data and materials notwithstanding, cross-national comparison remains and important analytical orientation in STS. Particularly with regard to the governance of biomedicine, biotechnology and the life sciences in a general sense, STS researchers have sought to make sense of differences—and to substantiate the idea that the current shape of science and technology is not a thing of necessity—through comparison. Often, such comparative research explores variability in science and technology (governance) by taking the nation state as its stable analytical unit (see, e.g., Daemmrich, 2004; Parthasarathy, 2007, 2017; Salter et al., 2016; Aarden, 2016). Framing differences between countries in terms of (techno)political cultures, much of this work focuses on the governance of novel technologies to understand how science and technology are culturally embedded and evaluated (Jasanoff, 2005; Felt et al., 2010). As Sheila Jasanoff (2005, p. 15) maintains, "comparison should be seen as a means of investigating the interactions between science and politics, with far-reaching implications for governance in advanced industrial democracies". In most cases, cross-national comparison in STS does not say a lot about border-crossing trajectories of research and technology development and how these are not only shaped by (national) idiosyncrasies, but also by asymmetrical geopolitical relations (Prasad, 2014a, b). Particularly in efforts to understand similarities, entanglements and differences between individual research initiatives, we thus need to move beyond comparisons presuming (largely) stable nation-states.[3]

The expanding cross-national trajectories of people, ideas and objects in science that increasingly position "the global inside the national" (Sassen, 2010) are not the only challenge for approaching comparison on the basis of largely static national cultures. In his book on environmental politics in Hong Kong, Timothy Choy (2011) traces how comparison is also an actor's category. In his work, comparison emerges as a rhetorical instrument used by activists to argue for particular forms of governance. Their use of comparison oscillates between arguments that either stress the uniqueness and specificity of Hong Kong, or position it in a universal narrative of environmental threats. Such differentiated deployment of comparison resonates with the interchanging local and global rhetorics surrounding medical research collections. They are not only legitimated with reference to national strengths and global relevance, but often crafted around arguments that involve and move across multiple scales. For example, the Framingham Heart Study mobilizes its location in a local community to advance the argument that it has and continues to contribute significant advances to medical research globally. Likewise, the Asian character of Singapore's population and a presumed tradition of sample collection in European welfare states are two different registers to pull from when arguing for a biobank in (a) particular location(s). All cases are thus rhetorically linked to specific locations while simultaneously performing their relevance at other scales.

To understand these particular multiscale dynamics of not only the rhetoric surrounding medical research, but also its practices of circulation, the trap of methodological nationalism (Wimmer & Schiller, 2003; Sassen, 2010), in which the nation-state is presumed to be an evident unit of analysis, should therefore be avoided. To be sure, the aim of helping address specific concerns regarding health or other social values are part of state-building processes in each of these cases—in addressing a major public health issue and helping shape a newly emerging national medical research system in the United States, pursuing a new "pillar" for the national economy in Singapore, repairing deficiencies in civil registration and public health in India, and integrating and harmonizing medical research in Europe. But none of these state-building activities can be reduced to the national scale. National concerns related to health inform these initiatives but never determine their shape. All of them overflow the national in order to build the state, not least due to the entanglements between building the state and pursuing specific areas of medical research that are not bound to national borders. As discussed above, none of these cases have an exclusively national referent and all of them are, in one way or another tied into broader scientific networks. Medical research involving these infrastructures thus moves between scales, but also creates and locates these particular scales (e.g., the global South in the Million Death Study or Europe in BBMRI-ERIC) in the process.

These somewhat nebulous and constantly shifting relations between different scales of imagination and practice within infrastructures for the purpose of population-based medical research affect how we may think and do comparison with such cases. They imply that comparison is never self-evident. All comparison is situated, raising the question what is made to be comparable and how (Deville et al., 2016). Jörg Niewöhner und Thomas Scheffer (2010, p. 4) bring this to the point when they write how "[o]bjects of comparison are not found 'out there' […] They are produced through *thickening* contextualisations, including analytical, cross-contextual framings that are meant to facilitate comparison". All comparison is both selective in its focus and reductive in the (limited) degree of complexity included. Comparison therefore requires the analyst to account for their analytical choices and contextualize their analysis. Along those lines, Michael Fischer (2018, p. 272) proposes a strategy of juxtaposition, which he sees as "a tactic of not abstracting from context […] while yet being able to gain a perspective on similarities and differences that may open up new ways of doing things in the varied local sites". Fischer applies this idea of juxtaposition to contrast how two Asian genome institutes, located in Singapore and Beijing respectively, are both situated locally and entangled in global professional and knowledge production networks. As an analytical strategy, juxtaposition can thereby avoid essentializing moves regarding where these institutes are, while still allowing for insights into their specific similarities and differences.

Taking the lead from Fischer's strategy while heeding the calls for accountability engrained in the notion of thick comparison, I propose that juxtaposing the four infrastructures I have analysed here allows for two different analytical moves. The first move is to conceptualize similarities and differences in how medical population research is presently done, with 'doing' including the whole range of institutional, technical, epistemic and other threads that make research infrastructures, which are inseparably knotted together. This is the move I made in this chapter, which allowed me to position these infrastructures in relation to some widely discussed developments in medical research (including datafication and capitalization of science, among others) and suggests that the infrastructures share the general thrust of these developments, but articulate them each in their own way. The other move concerns my normative agenda in writing this, which is to scrutinize claims towards medical research as an unassailable good by unravelling and indeed juxtaposing the normative commitments built into medical research collections. I attend to these by deploying the notion of citizenship as an analytical lens in the next, concluding chapter.

Conclusion: Positioning Medical Research Infrastructures

In this chapter, I have drawn insights from the previously presented cases together to further develop my analytical heuristic of infrastructures for the purpose of population-based medical research. I here described infrastructures as simultaneously functional and imaginative constructs that allow for the circulation of research materials and ideas; purposes as imaginaries of the value of research that get realized (or not) through the active construction and contestation of value; populations as entities that get constructed, fragmented and reconstructed through the generation and classification of data; and medical research as an amalgam of practices and institution in which particular pathways for constructing knowledge are negotiated. I subsequently argued that this analytical heuristic foregrounds how such infrastructures may be understood as sociomaterial, multiple, imaginative and situated. Through these descriptors, I sought to capture the volatility of infrastructures in spite of their seeming robustness. In other words, their meaning is always negotiable and shaped according to specific circumstances, which suggests that no singular, persistent identity can be attributed to any medical research collection (see also Radin, 2013, 2014). They surely restrict how medical research can be done, but these restrictions are a matter of choices and practices that can also be altered. That said, as phenomena located in the present I also considered how these infrastructures are positioned in relation to, and in various ways reflect trends towards state-making, bioeconomies, new social contracts for science and big data that characterize contemporary research. While these cases are all different, they also embody significant similarities.

I further thought through these similarities and differences by addressing the methodological purchase of comparison in relation to the increasingly international or global networks of science. While I see limited value for these cases in focusing on cross-national comparison that presumes these infrastructures to be reflections of national (techno)political cultures, I see value in a more dynamic strategy of 'thicker' comparison and juxtaposition. Such a strategy would not only imply to attend to both situational specificities and connections beyond specific locations. It also invites explicit reflection on the choices made and the commitments that inform comparative analysis.

To come full circle to the opening of this book, I therefore return to the presumed public good of medical knowledge and participation in medical research in the conclusion. The formula that people have a moral obligation to participate in medical research because it produces generalizable medical knowledge (Owen Schaefer et al., 2009) postulates a generic notion of rights and responsibilities. I interrogate this postulate by approaching rights and responsibilities in terms of biological and social citizenship through a juxtaposition of the four case studies. My aim is to use citizenship as a lens to zoom in on the distinct ways rights and responsibilities relative to health get defined. That different configurations of citizenship may be distilled from these cases implies that a more careful approach to the question of participation is needed. We cannot presume a blanket obligation to participate if the (indirect) benefits of participation take substantially different shapes. Furthermore, so Richard Tutton (2007) has indicated, participation in medical research collections (or biobanks) has an ambivalent dual meaning that includes participation *in research* as a research subject and *in the governance of research*. This second notion of participation has been widely discussed in the ethical literature on biobanking and in the social science literature on the governance of science and technology. I touch on these discussions, but will argue that this kind of participation (also described as engagement) cannot provide a *sufficient* response to the political questions contemporary medical research collections pose. A broader approach to citizenship and democracy in relation to health is therefore needed.

Notes

1. Another way to describe infrastructures for the purpose of population-based medical research may thus be in terms of material-semiotics (Law, 2009). This is also implied by using the term "to do" here, which draws on notions such as performativity and enactment that are central to this perspective. I do not adopt this terminology, however, since I want to maintain that some of the institutional environments within which these infrastructures are established (of e.g., the state) are more resistant to such doings (or, in other word, limit the range of options) more strongly than even Law's (2004) notion of "hinterlands", which seems to try to address this issue, would allow for.
2. For a similar discussion regarding the various meanings of big data, see (Ward & Barker, 2013).
3. It is worth noting how this assumption can be analytically and politically problematic. In many ways, for example, the financial crisis of 2008 had repercussions on European countries that make it questionable whether—or to what degree—these were still "the same" countries. It remains to be seen what the radical destruction of the administrative state in the United States as part of the second, Trump presidency will mean for its "political culture" as well. I thank Alessandro Blasimme for our discussion on this point many years ago.

7

Revisiting Medical Research Participation Through Citizenship

I opened this book with a critical discussion of the claim that all of us may be expected to participate in or donate materials for medical research, since it supplies the public good of generalizable medical knowledge (Owen Schaefer et al., 2009). While this idea, and its inherent assumption that access to medical knowledge is unproblematic in particular, has been critically received (Rennie, 2011), the idea nevertheless appears to have staying power, for example in relation to more recent areas of medical innovation in, for example, artificial intelligence (Müller, 2022). Moreover, the idea that obstacles to widespread use of tissue and data should be removed as much as possible is also central to ethical notions of 'broad' or 'blanket' consent (Rothstein, 2005; Otlowski, 2009; Smilan, 2022) and calls for widespread sharing of materials (Stark et al., 2025). All of these claims that presume medical knowledge to be what economists might call a non-rivalrous public good (equally available to all without diminishing), however, share a "view from nowhere" on medical research. Yet, as Donna Haraway (1991) has famously argued, such a view obscures how all knowledge (production) is "situated", shaped by the particular circumstances of production and positionality of its producers. Scientific research thereby (re)produces social inequalities and asymmetries both in its ways of knowing and in how and to whom

E. Aarden, *Producing Citizenship in Medical Research Collections*, Health, Technology and Society, https://doi.org/10.1007/978-981-95-1707-7_7

knowledge is accessible (Harding, 2006). Informed by these perspectives, I therefore focused on the coproduction (Jasanoff, 2004) of research practices, science governance and ways of knowing health and disease in population-based medical research collections, with an eye on how particular forms of knowledge (can) benefit particular 'publics'.

In four case studies of medical research collections located in India, Singapore, the United States and across Europe and focusing on different areas of medical research that range from genomics and chronic disease epidemiology to global health,[1] I have proposed the notion of *infrastructures for the purpose of population-based medical research* as an analytical heuristic. I used this heuristic to show the complex and volatile configuration of medical research collections while simultaneously showing how particular sociomaterial configurations and imaginations of research shaped research purposes and outcomes. I used these observations to argue that my cases partially reflect current trends in medical research, but also how such broadly diagnosed trends manifest in particular ways in distinct situations. To attend to those specificities and to account for their normative implications, I took on the idea of "thick" comparison (Niewöhner & Scheffer, 2010), which invites analysts to make their own decisions and commitments in comparison explicit.

In this chapter, I take these ideas on board to further develop my discussion of the intersections between meanings of health and disease and individual and collective rights and responsibilities in tissue and data collections for medical research. I first move to a discussion of citizenship in the context of medical research. I use this notion as an analytical lens that allows me to zoom in on how rights and responsibilities get defined in medical research collections. I therefore begin by positioning claims concerning the emergence of new, biology-based forms of citizenship in a wider discourse on citizenship transformations, before teasing out how the biological and the social jointly shape citizenship in my case studies. On the basis of that analysis, I return to and expand the discussion on research participation. Considering the ambivalent nature of participation in both research and research governance in and of biobanks (Tutton, 2007), I engage with questions of what I would rather call public engagement in biobanks (Overby et al., 2015) and science and technology governance more broadly (Irwin, 2015; Chilvers & Kearnes, 2016). Since I consider the issues at stake to extend beyond research participation, I take these discussions as a starting point for considering broader questions of science and democracy in conclusion.

Citizenship Formations in Medical Research Collections

So far, I have developed an analysis of practices and governance of data and tissue collections for medical research. Conceptualizing collections as infrastructures for the purpose of population-based medical research, I have traced the entanglements between broader organizational, regulatory and financial formations, relations and materiality in scientific work and (where applicable) the formulation and use of particular research questions, methods of data collection and analysis, and resulting knowledge claims. I thereby engaged with literature on the promises and practices of medical research collections, arguing that the meanings of such collections are situated yet multiple and contested, and intersect with broader trends in medical research.

In this section, I want to pick up on the distinction Herbert Gottweis and Alan Petersen (2008) have made between governance *of* and governance *through* biobanks and relate to discussions of justice in relation to scientific and technological projects (Mamo & Fishman, 2013). I do so through a discussion of the rights and responsibilities—which I capture under the notion citizenship—that are generated through efforts to collect, store, exchange and use tissue and data for medical research. I align this discussion with broader debates on contemporary citizenship and will attend to rights and responsibilities for both individuals and collectives, but also in relation to research participants as well as presumed wider collectives of (potential) beneficiaries.

The notion that developments in the (bio)medical sciences can have consequences for individual and collective rights and responsibilities rests on perspectives on governance in terms of biopolitics and biopower. The latter term, introduced and defined by Michel Foucault (2007, p. 1) as "the set of mechanisms through which the basic biological features of the human species became the object of [...] a general strategy of power" describes how knowledge about (human) life turned such life into an object of political intervention (see also Lemke, 2007). While Foucault mainly focused on the emergence of the notion of population and the use of statistics in government, more recent theorists of biopower have argued that "the biological existence of human beings has become political in novel ways" (Rose, 2001, p. 1) in conjunction with changing scientific views of life. Thus, the emergence of molecular biology, medical focus on disease risks and understandings of health in terms of quality of life have contributed to the emergence of new form of governance (Rabinow & Rose, 2006; Wahlberg & Rose, 2015).

Such emerging, new (molecular) forms of biopower have also been theorized as sources of new kinds of social collectives that neither resemble traditional 'population' nor are primarily defined by the state (Rabinow, 2005; Rabinow & Rose, 2006; Hacking, 2006). Carlos Novas and Nikolas Rose (2000) have famously described how, particularly in relation to the emergence of genetic understandings of life and health, a new kind of individual personhood has developed. They describe this personhood in terms of a somatic individual who is defined in terms of genetic risk for disease. This type of risk, so Novas and Rose, has resulted in the formation of new kinds of collectives and a novel sense of (genetic) responsibility. Elsewhere, they describe transformations in responsibilities and (claims to) rights as biological citizenship (Rose & Novas, 2005), arguing that new developments in the life sciences give rise to citizenship claims from below, on a genetic basis (see also Heath et al., 2008). Such bottom-up conceptions of biological citizenship are based on particular assumptions about social identities and rationalities that may give rise to claims to rights and resources on a biological basis (Johnson et al., 2018). However, other notions of citizenship based in biological characteristics do consider claims to be made towards and attributed by the state (Petryna, 2004; Cooter, 2008). The notion of biological citizenship thereby raises the question how and by whom rights and responsibilities are reframed in relation to specific ways of knowing and defining life (Jasanoff, 2011; Hurlbut et al., 2020).

Beyond the question what role remains for the state, some of the more influential formulations of biological citizenship have been critiqued on the basis of a set of foundational assumptions about biology, citizenship rights and social order (see also Aarden, 2018). First, critics have argued that the relation between the molecular, the individual and population is more complex than assumed in the notion of biological citizenship. Not only are the medical sciences (still) far from defining all diseases in genetic terms, genetics also relies significantly on established categories of population and race, gender and even class to identify human difference (Raman & Tutton, 2010; Kowal, 2022; Roberts & Tutton, 2018). Furthermore, in spite of claims about citizenship claims arising bottom up from new collectives, some critics emphasize the institutional dimension of allocating rights, responsibilities and resources. Often, the state and other public institutions remain important in determining which claims have merit—particularly in the context of medical science and technology (Benjamin, 2013). As a result, the unequal distribution of health-related resources (beyond innovative medical technology alone) is often based on a set of institutional logics and routines that are based on many more considerations than one's genetic profile alone. Thus, "to prioritise the biological is often *ipso facto* to produce a reductive account of problems, solutions, and identities" (Plows & Boddington, 2006, p. 119). Moreover, to presume a generic 'biological' basis to citizenship obscures how global inequalities can produce embodied health effects, thus reshaping the biology supposedly underlying citizenship itself (Sparke, 2017). Along with questioning the lack of attention to the complexity and multiplicity of life and citizenship, critics thereby also suggest that a focus on biological risks and characteristics might obscure other factors that shape the distribution of citizenship rights and responsibilities.

Nevertheless, biology, knowledge and citizenship are historically linked, as for example suggested through the related notion of health citizenship (Jauho & Helén, 2023). This conceptualization of citizenship focuses on populations' biological characteristics in relation to membership in a collective, individual rights and responsibilities and questions of participation. This perspective on biology or vitality in the context of citizenship seeks to "provide a perspective on how biological and medical facts and related expert knowledge enter in and influence the domains in which citizenship is defined and struggled over" (Jauho & Helén, 2023, p. 469). This concept thereby suggests a deeper connection between citizenship and the facts of life, mediated through institutions. It thereby invites a reading of citizenship discourses that is both attentive to the historical emergence of citizenship as a political category, while simultaneously foregrounding its implications for individual and collective notions of health.

The notion of health citizenship suggests that citizenship is not exclusively about biology, even though it is always also about biology. This perspective invites a particular reading of contemporary citizenship discourse in relation to medical research repositories. Much recent work on citizenship has observed how the meaning of citizenship has always been contested and subject to transformation (Pfister, 2012; Kivisto & Faist, 2007; Heater, 2004). Even the seemingly self-evident contemporary link between citizenship and the nation-state only emerged in the nineteenth century. At present, this presumed link is under increasing pressure, along with the idea that citizenship involves a gradual expansion of rights (Magnette, 2005; Takle et al., 2023). While citizenship may be said to describe—in both an analytical and moral register—relations between the individual and the collective (Faulks, 2000), it remains subject to negotiation what this collective is and what such relations entail. In particular, contested dimensions of citizenship at this time revolve around notions of the decreased relevance of the nation state and national belonging, a presumed decline in participation in public life and an erosion of social citizenship that includes access to public resources (Kivisto & Faist, 2007).

The historical development of citizenship is often described as a progressive story, involving the expansion of citizenship from basic civil and political rights to the notion of social citizenship that includes a redistribution of social resources (Heater, 2004; Magnette, 2005; Revi, 2014). The notion of social citizenship is of particular interest since it has been argued to form a precondition for the 'true' realization of civil and political rights (Heater, 2004; Laruffa, 2022), but has also been understood in opposition to them. Moreover, the notion central to social citizenship that citizenship can be about "access to societal resources" (Pfister, 2012, p. 26) appears increasingly uncertain with the widely discussed decline of the welfare state, which, some observers have suggested, cannot be seen separate from arguments in favour of research and innovation as a public good that circumvents the need for addressing structural social and economic inequalities (Reardon, 2017; Benjamin, 2013). These observations beg the question if and how participation in medical research collections is framed in relation to social citizenship understood in terms of access to collective resources and services.

Various other supposed transformations in the meaning of citizenship and associated rights and responsibilities may feature into medical research collections, beyond the question of social rights (see also Kivisto & Faist, 2007; Wohlfarth, 2020). The decline of social citizenship rights also raises questions about the (often implicit) expectation that citizens participate in public life, as a retreating welfare state may also leave citizens to question the grounds for contributing to collective affairs (Kivisto & Faist, 2007). Furthermore, the loosening link between citizenship and the nation-state seems relevant, not only in terms of the outsourcing of welfare to research and innovation (cf. Petryna, 2004), but also in light of the growing emphasis on cross-border circulation of tissue and data, which problematizes any nationalized understanding of the benefits of science (Cool, 2016). In sum, a discussion of citizenship requires thinking of medical research collections not only as machineries for knowledge production, but also social and political institutions that affect if and how health is defined as an issue of collective concern.

Debates about an alleged decline in social citizenship rights and associated decrease in active political participation as well as those concerning citizenship detaching from the nation-state (Magnette, 2005; Revi, 2014) thus present the background against which citizenship may be used as an analytical lens for medical research collections. In particular, taking these discourses into account in an analysis of citizenship moves beyond the biological in research collections to also consider how declining participation, reorientation of social rights and the changing locus of citizenship feature into the inscription of rights and responsibilities in research infrastructures. Aihwa Ong (2006a), for example, has argued that the uncoupling of citizenship from the nation-state has made new and expanded grounds on which to claim citizenship possible, while simultaneously making citizens themselves responsible for their well-being. Moreover, such shifts work out differently in different places.

These various transformations in the location and content of citizenship then raise the question how citizenship allows an analytic focused on the framing of individual and collective rights and responsibilities through participation in medical research collections that accounts for both biological and social dimensions. I explore this issue by returning to the case studies and reconsidering them along three dimensions I draw from the citizenship literature. First, I take a cue from the literature on biological citizenship to consider which *biological* characteristics and forms of knowledge are central to the allocation of rights and responsibilities. Second, I bring these into conversation with understandings of citizenship in terms of membership to consider the *collectives* formed by and in relation to specific (state) institutions. Third, I engage with discourses on the decline of citizenship to address both the kinds of (social) *rights* included and how these relate to expectations—or *responsibilities*—of participation.

Framingham Heart Study

The focus of the Framingham Heart Study has been on identifying the "coronary prone individual" (Kannel et al., 1961), which has by and large been framed in terms of individual behavioural risk factors. From the beginning of the study onwards, risk has been defined by correlating certain lifestyle traits (as well as some other characteristics) to the occurrence of a particular list of cardiovascular conditions. This is the essence of the risk factor concept and of the prospective epidemiological method supposedly piloted by the Framingham Heart Study. The biology of cardiovascular disease and ways of knowing it are thereby reduced to a very particular logic of cause and effect. Remarkably, this logic was largely maintained once new—not least of all genetic—approaches to disease emerged. Even now, the risk factor remains largely individual and linked to lifestyle. Genetic predispositions then only add more urgency to the need to change behaviour. Nevertheless, and despite challenges emerging from its long duration, the study has engaged with many novel research methods and techniques. In the process, other aspects of study participants' biology beyond their behaviour have gained significance. For example, the sequential data and blood samples that go back decades have made the study's resources into a repository that can help answer questions other studies cannot. As a result, Framingham Heart Study participants' biology has become a research object in ever new ways.

Despite the changing status of participants' biology, one of the distinctive properties of the study is its persistent understanding of their collectivity. From the initial recruitment of participants to the present, the Framingham Heart Study is both externally presented and internally understood as a community-based study. Particular aspects of the local community drew the interest of study initiators and today its ties to the community are still understood as one of the main strengths of the study. It is, for example, tied into another important form of collective considered important in allowing the study to work as it does, which is the notion of families. (Biological) family relations are considered important for the particular forms of research they allow—particularly around the heritability of disease. Yet these notions of community and family obscure particular implications and exclusions that characterize the study. Although Framingham has been touted as a "typically American" town (Gehlbach, 2005), there are structural racial biases in its initial population sample which, at least in that sense, was not at all representative of the United States (Shim, 2014).[2] At the same time, the heavy reliance on community engagement contributed to the exclusion of certain hypotheses of social determinants of health from the initial study. Furthermore, the study's prominence results to a meaningful degree from its position within the overall 'portfolio' of epidemiological research projects funded and administered by the NIH. The Framingham Heart Study was hence initiated and delivered its first, most consequential, insights in parallel to and as part of the establishment of the American post-War public research landscape.

Through its particular focus on individual lifestyle risks, the Framingham Heart Study has contributed to an understanding of health in terms of responsibilities rather than rights. In fact, one can find statements lamenting the lack of lifestyle changes in response to the study's insights in various writings from study personnel (Dawber, 1980; Levy & Brink, 2005). This is all the more remarkable in relation to Anne Pollock's (2012) observation that, in the equivalent Jackson Heart Study focusing on African-Americans, socioeconomic hypotheses have been investigated. Considering these two studies in contrast suggests that different *kinds of* health risks—and thereby different rights and responsibilities—are considered along racial lines and thereby maintain racial inequalities. In addition, framing cardiovascular disease in terms of lifestyle risks that can be corrected (Kannel, 1987; Kannel & Wilson, 2007) has had far reaching consequences for modern framings of public health and citizenship in terms of individual responsibility (Aronowitz, 1998; Rothstein, 2003; Giroux, 2013). Against this background, the Framingham Heart Study is not only an influential example of how health and health risks have been defined since the second half of the twentieth century, but also of how such definitions resonate with particular institutional configurations and distributions of rights and responsibilities in relation to (individual) biology (Aarden, 2018). This, in turn, raises further questions about if and how knowledge that locates responsibility with the individual can or cannot be considered a *public* good.

Singapore Tissue Network

The distinctive biological feature of people (indirectly) participating or donating tissue and data to the Singapore Tissue Network is how one nation's population came to stand in as biologically representative for an entire continent (Ong, 2013, 2015). The 'Asian' character of the population's classification into Chinese, Indian and Malay groups was not only rhetorically mobilized to argue for medical research in Singapore. It simultaneously was a factor in recruiting participants, both in studies focusing on specific population groups and in matching recruiters with desired participants. However, since the Singapore Tissue Network did not itself recruit participants or collect samples, Asian representativeness was not a criterion for the collection as such. In terms of the STN collection, the focus was on getting different researchers receiving national research grants to centrally store their materials and thereby make them available for others to use. What was of biological interest in the STN was hence what was of interest in individual research projects. Adjacently, the focus in knowledge production was on how to facilitate collaboration in research rather than on addressing any specific research questions. This entailed particular presumptions of how science works, which we have seen to conflict with practising scientists' imaginations of how to collaborate in research—a conflict that crystallized in the separation of samples and data.

This separation is possibly the lasting image of how a collective of research subjects was formed in STN storage. It was largely an imaginary collective, both in terms of how the separation of tissue and data was imagined to serve productivity, but also in how no collective of research participants materialized beyond a rather elusive notion of Singapore citizens or patients making materials available for research. Nevertheless, the particular institutional configuration of and around the Singapore Tissue Network ties to a more distinct imaginary of how the collective would benefit from research. The network was established as a support facility for investments in biomedical research that were initiated by a combination of government agencies that jointly saw economic potential in the biomedical sciences. As I have observed, this logic reflected a foundational imaginary in Singapore that social stability and progress depend on economic growth pursued in subsequently more advanced scientific and technological domains (Low, 2004; Trocki, 2009). This particular legitimation strategy for the state's proactive role in economic development was also linked to imagining benefits for Singapore's population. Although not formally perceived as redistributive policies, the government in Singapore has long invested economic gains in, for example, public housing, health care and other public services (Mutalib, 2004; Chua, 2005; Reisman, 2009). Although this notion of collective benefit was not referenced explicitly in relation to medical tissue and data repositories in Singapore, much about the Biomedical Sciences Initiative suggests that it continued to pursue this particular logic of making the fruits of economic development available to the population.

Rights and responsibilities related to tissue storage in the Singapore Tissue Network hence remain largely implicit and indirect. Participation in research may possibly be seen as a contribution to knowledge production and economic growth—and indeed some of the social science literature in biomedical research in Singapore suggests that there were active attempts to enrol citizens in medical research (Holden & Demeritt, 2008;

Waldby, 2009b). Yet the focus on research collaboration in the Singapore Tissue Network operated at a different level, aiming to provide support for high-quality storage and sharing of biological materials. Nevertheless, we do find particular concern with sample donors and research participants at individual research institutes or decentral biobanks that directly recruit and collect. Particularly in the context of epidemiological studies, my exploration of participant recruitment suggests that donors are treated as more than mere contributors of research materials. More precisely, I found that care for the elderly was performed in various ways in recruitment. While my interview respondent was clear about ultimately wanting a person to contribute blood samples and data and not to prematurely terminate their engagement with the research team, this also required providing a number of services and small gestures. These ranged from building trust in the recruitment process, arranging transport, food and beverages as part of the examination, to recommending further medical attention when needed. In some cases, so the suggestion, research participation then becomes a stand-in for regular care not because health care services are not available (see, e.g., Cooper & Waldby, 2014), but out of a seeming sense of responsibility towards research participants.

Million Death Study

The focus in the Million Death Study is on the distribution of causes of death in the population, which are identified through a particular approach to knowledge production centred on the verbal autopsy method. The particular way the biological characteristics of the Indian population are thereby captured informs the important—yet, so the argument of study researchers as well as many others goes, also neglected (Global Health Watch, 2011; Drèze & Sen, 2013; Economic and Political Weekly, 2015)—social domain of public health. Since part of this neglect takes the form of insufficient registration of causes of death, parsing what causes people to die is the issue of biological interest here. To answer this question, knowledge production mobilizes the representative demographic sample of the SRS and applies the verbal autopsy method to any death in this sample. This method implies a fragmentation of individual mortality, since each death is deconstructed into descriptions of a set and sequence of symptoms in a household interview. These symptomatic data points are put back together in physicians' efforts to arrive at a diagnosis, and individual diagnoses are in turn aggregated to describe death in India at both national and regional levels on the basis of specific, medically classified causes. Researchers acknowledge that these statistics have limitations, since not all medical conditions can be distinguished based on verbal descriptions and none of the causes of death have been clinically confirmed. Nevertheless, the representativeness of the sample is seen as decisive for researchers' conviction that MDS statistics are more reliable than formal government mortality data.

Central to the Million Death Study is thereby an understanding of the population as a collective that is underserved by existing public knowledge infrastructures and, as a consequence, public health institutions. This understanding involves a paradoxical relation to the state. On the one hand, deficiencies of the state in the domain of health form a key motivation for the study. At the same time, the study is not conceived as an (academic) research project but integrated into a different state infrastructure, that of the Registrar General's Office responsible for the census and the SRS. Consequently, the study needs the state as an alternative to the state, while being simultaneously tied into a global health network of government and research institutions in India, but also in the global North. Study coordination, data analysis and funding all are located both in India and elsewhere (and involve both non-Indian state institutions such as the NIH and non-state institutions such as the Gates Foundation, both of which finance certain parts of the study). Moreover, the study ultimately ties back to the Indian state's responsibilities in the health domain as well, as findings from the MDS are expected to contribute to improved health policy-making. In this process, the population collective is not only conceived in terms of mortality or as ultimate beneficiaries of mortality statistics (a point I return to below). The SRS sample, which in classic statistical fashion is supposed to stand in for the population of India as a whole, simultaneously models for a much wider collective, which is the population of the global South. Not only do initiators of the Million Death Study suggest that the *method* of verbal autopsy could be applied in other low resource settings, they simultaneously claim that by virtue of the highly uneven distribution of causes of death, study *findings* bear relevance for populations elsewhere, too.

The Million Death Study is thereby based on the presumption that motivating relatives of people who have died to tell a careful story about the circumstances of death, or—put differently—that asking the right questions can provide representative and accurate enough "estimates" of the causal distribution of mortality in a population. On this basis, their associated claim is that such insight can be used to improve public health policy and thus reduce premature death from certain causes. This presumption is sometimes based on what seems to be a somewhat oversimplified conception of the policy process, as I illustrated with the example of shifting funds from the HIV/AIDS programme to anti-snake venom if deaths from the former appear to be less and from the latter more common than previously thought. Yet such ideas notwithstanding, there are more elaborate notions of how mortality insights may be translated into health policy change (Jha & Laxminarayan, 2009). However, a shared characteristics of the public 'impact' of the Million Death Study appears to be that improvements in public health can be framed in terms of interventions tailored to specific diseases. This in spite of well-established research on the social determinants of health (Cockerham, 2013; Marmot, 2015) and calls for basic healthcare and more structural interventions as preconditions for improving the mortality profile of India's population (Rao, 2001; Rao et al., 2015). Within the Million Death Study, citizens' rights and responsibilities with regard to health instead appear to be conceived in a relatively narrow sense.

BBMRI-ERIC

The approach to sample collection and storage in BBMRI-ERIC is to some degree similar to the Singapore Tissue Network. It also does not involve a specific recruitment or collection strategy—at least not at the European level—but, in contrast to the STN, there is also no centralized sample storage. The biological characteristics of concern and the research questions asked in relation to BBMRI-ERIC are thus defined at the level of individual research institutions and biobanks. Biological characteristics of the materials and data distributed in BBMRI-ERIC then matter in how they are represented in the Directory, which serves the purpose of allowing researchers to find materials that would be of interest for them to work with. Yet here, too, the role of BBMRI-ERIC's central administration is limited, since individual biobanks decide which exact data on their collections they share in the Directory. Knowledge production that makes use of materials from BBMRI-ERIC member biobanks can take a wide variety of forms and involve a wide range of biological characteristics of the individual donors. Nevertheless, BBMRI-ERIC does refer to certain, if mostly implicit aspects of a European population that is made available for research through the repository. At the same time, the idea that BBMRI-ERIC provides access to biological materials from all around Europe is not without its problems, as some people observed that the infrastructure has perhaps not been as successful in advancing sample exchange as desired (not to mention that contributions are very unevenly distributed in Europe).

Still, more than in the comparatively similar Singapore Tissue Network, European citizens and institutions form a relatively explicit point of reference. On the one hand, BBMRI-ERIC is argued to have built this rather complex infrastructure for the citizens of Europe, to improve their medical care and supply them with new treatments. On the other hand, the argument particularly at the beginning has been that a European biobanking infrastructure can be built with existing collections because there had already been a 'European' tradition of collection in the context of state health services. However, this European tradition appears to have been located in a relatively limited number of, primarily Nordic, countries (Tupasela et al., 2020). More generally, the category of Europe is a challenging notion for and within BBMRI-ERIC. The infrastructure can be read as an effort to institutionalize Europe in the biomedical research domain, both building on European Union efforts in science policy and confronting certain entrenched challenges of making Europe. European policy strategies (ESFRI), regulations (ERIC) and project funding have been vital for bringing BBMRI-ERIC into existence. At the same time, the logic of the ERIC legal framework, as well as European integration writ large (Ryan, 2021) entails ongoing recalibration of common European interests and initiatives with member state claims to subsidiarity. This balancing act is further complicated in BBMRI-ERIC by the membership of individual biobanks (as part of member state National Nodes). All this implies not only that the European collective is often highly uncertain, but also that making a European collective is what the infrastructure is (supposed to be) working towards.

The uncertain and contested aims of BBMRI-ERIC, which range from participating in research to the delivery of support services and from scientific ambitions to enabling innovation for the market, also mean that it remains nebulous what citizens may expect from the infrastructure. Citizens thereby remain at a relative distance from BBMRI-ERIC, only engaging with individual local biobanks or national infrastructures at best. BBMRI-ERIC is supposed to lay the groundwork—to build the infrastructure, if you will—for the operation of individual biobanks and research institutions. It intends to do so by, for example, harmonizing procedures, developing standards, making materials visible and assessing the quality of potential collaboration partners. To be sure, none of these things directly affect the rights and responsibilities of individual citizens or patients and all of them are fairly uncertain in light of the complexity of European collaboration in research. BBMRI-ERIC is ultimately in the business of European integration with all its complexities and paradoxes. The ultimate aim of this is to improve medicine and health for the citizens of Europe, so representatives of BBMRI-ERIC maintain. Yet the question remains if and how complex, multi-layered infrastructures can contribute to resolving the alleged "paradox" that European science fails to deliver successful (technological) applications.[3]

In this section, I used citizenship as an analytical lens to uncover how data and tissue collections for medical research entail particular normative commitments and, more precisely, how they attribute certain rights and responsibilities to both individual and collective participants and wider publics. It turned out that not all of them do so equally explicitly along each of these dimensions. I would maintain that this is in part due to the particular 'situations' in and for which data and tissue get collected. By this I mean that my case studies include both more or less specific projects (even if longitudinal ones) oriented towards specific research aims and questions and infrastructures or support structures for which the research aims are more fragmented and diffuse. This matters for how citizenship may be formulated.

That said, each of these cases navigates particular notions of biological characteristics and forms of knowledge that matter, particular relations between collectives and institutions and particular allocations of rights and responsibilities (see Table 7.1). Yet, what I find across these cases is a relatively limited orientation towards particular forms of social rights and citizenship pertaining to health (Jauho & Helén, 2023). I characterized rights and responsibilities as individualized in the context of the Framingham Heart Study, implicit and indirect for the Singapore Tissue Network, narrowly biomedical in the Million Death Study and distant in BBMRI-ERIC. While these are admittedly rather superficial characterizations (and I do not wish to capture citizenship in single terms), they jointly suggest that tissue and data collection efforts for medical research reflect the broader trend of biomedicalization (Clarke et al., 2010). In particular, other non-medical dimensions of health, including the relational and material characteristics of its social dimensions (cf. Yates-Doerr, 2020) receive less consideration. This implies that medical research collections, in spite of the multitudes of samples and data on virtually all (biological) aspects of life they can contain, cannot be the only answer to the question how to care for human health. This brings me back to the multiple meanings of participation, which I will address in conclusion.

Participation and the Democratization of Science

Participation in medical research (collections) has a dual meaning, referring both to contributions as a research subject or donor of tissue or data and to engagement in the governance of research (Tutton, 2007). In the literature on biobanking ethics, these two meanings often intersect. Participation in governance is then presented as a means to build public trust, which, in turn, is said to be a prerequisite for research participation (Overby et al., 2015; Adjekum et al., 2017). Many ethicists have therefore argued in favour of public engagement and participation in the

Table 7.1 Citizenship in four infrastructures for the purpose of population-based medical research

	FHS	STN	MDS	BBMRI-ERIC
Biology and knowledge	Epidemiology of individual CVD risks	Asian representativeness in individual studies	Cause of death statistics captured with verbal autopsy	Determined in individual biobanks and research institutes
Collectives and institutions	Community and families in national portfolio	Population as imagined beneficiaries of growth through state institutions	Underserved population; reorienting state in global health networks	European citizens; complexity of European integration
Rights and responsibilities	Based on individual lifestyle	Implicit expectation of research participation; care in recruitment	Narrow biomedical framing of mortality	Distant contributors and beneficiaries in integrated European science

governance of research collections (McWhirter et al., 2014; Gaskell et al., 2013; Knoppers & Chadwick, 2005). Yet in spite of this wide recognition of the importance of donor engagement[4] some observers argue that in many cases, research institutions appear to "[embrace] the need for public engagement (if not the democratic principles behind it)" (Stranger & Kaye, 2009, p. 11). While public engagement thereby appears to provide a pathway for acquiescing some concerns about research participation, it is not clear if it provides a suitable answer for concerns citizens may have.

One reason why formal modes of engagement may not necessarily meet the needs of participants is that they often engage a "phantom public" (Gottweis et al., 2011). Participant engagement thereby seems to aim for avoiding public controversy rather than addressing any reservations (potential) participants may have about the purposes and implications of research. Formal approaches thereby often pursue a narrow notion of engagement and, by extension, of the kinds of social and political issues that medical research may raise (Cañada et al., 2015). Such approaches may thereby overlook how "[a] key issue [for biobank governance] is how a biobank socially constructs biobank participants, donors and citizens in a way that is compatible with its (macro)politics and cultural context" (Gottweis & Lauss, 2011, p. 68). Without attending to the political and cultural context, medical research collections risk not only loosing trust, but will also miss opportunities to more adequately address people's health related concerns. If (formal) public engagement is to improve the social acceptance of medical research collections, then, it should not only focus on participant identities, but also engage communities' perspectives and knowledges to make sure research is appropriate (Goisauf & Durnovà, 2019). Only when taking the dynamic and diverse possible contributions of participants seriously can engagement be truly helpful in advancing research that serves public health.

Yet the question then (still) remains whether participant engagement does justice to the ways medical research collections shape citizen rights and responsibilities. About four decades of public engagement research in STS suggests that this is a vexing question that requires a more fundamental discussion of the purposes and merits of public engagement (that should start with going beyond research participants alone). Theorists of public engagement with science and technology have long presented the so-called deficit model of the public as the fundamental but persistent problem in controversies around science and technology. This model implies a view of resistance or concern about science and technology as a matter of ignorance (Irwin, 2015). A central accusation levelled at the deficit model has consequently been its presumed undifferentiated view of both science and the public. General concern about public ignorance and scepticism towards science was often seen to be tied to limited attention for the quite specific stakes and meanings people attribute to particular fields of science or technological developments (Michael, 2009). In this context, formalized public engagement exercises have been accused of framing publics in such a way that engagement served as a mechanism for producing social acceptance of science and technology (Thorpe & Gregory, 2010). By contrast, more 'informal' affected and concerned publics have been found to emerge or gather around particular issues of concern (Marres, 2007). Work on public engagement in STS has thereby shown the many forms publics can take, the many ways they can engage and the wide variety of concerns regarding science and technology they may express (Chilvers & Kearnes, 2016).

In their various discussions of public engagement with science and technology, STS researchers have thereby consistently claimed that debates about science and technology are essentially more profound political debates about the appropriate role of technoscientific developments in society. Against that background, Brian Wynne (2006) has argued how public engagement often—to paraphrase a widely cited formulation—"hits the notes, but misses the music". He thereby stresses that public concerns about science are often misunderstood as being hostile to science, while they are in effect about how science and technology affect collective well-being. Public engagement in response often operates at too narrow a scale to do justice to the far-reaching social implications of public issues related to science and technology and the complex questions of governance they invoke (Stilgoe et al., 2014). This is why in the context of medical research collections engagement cannot just involve participants and why governance of medical research cannot just be about how to govern them. The politics of medical research (collections) need to be about why research is done as well and as such requires broader democratic procedures than 'mere' public engagement exercises.

Thinking through the democratization of medical research collections beyond participant engagement requires considering citizenship as a normative, rather than just analytical, category (cf. Magnette, 2005). As infrastructures that are claimed to generate medical knowledge accessible to all, it seems reasonable to approach such collections in terms of health citizenship. This notion can be understood as a concept for describing "the ways modern states have embraced ensuring the vitality and well-being of the population as their central task and transformed into welfare states" (Jauho & Helén, 2023, p. 469). However, as Francisco Laruffa (2022, p. 376) has noted, (social) citizenship cannot just be about social policy. In its ideal form, it "represents more than just a set of welfare benefits and services". For social citizenship to be truly realized, and to thereby give substance to civil and political citizenship as well, requires citizen's full participation in society through an extension of citizenship's democratic dimensions. Yet, in her work on the "postgenomic condition" Jenny Reardon expresses her doubts about the intersections of (in her case) genomic knowledge and democracy. She writes how "[r]ather than an emblematic public good, genomics today bears witness to the broader erosion of the meaning of the public as a domain that fosters consideration of common concerns and the creation of collective goods" (Reardon, 2017, p. 189). She thereby seems to postulate that the absence of public deliberation on the purposes of research eventually results in limited public value emerging from research. In genomics, so it seems, social citizenship includes neither democracy nor social policy.[5]

Taking the notion that democracy is a prerequisite for the full realization of social citizenship seriously consequently suggests the need to critically assess imaginaries of the benefits of science and innovation that "invoke citizens as the ultimate and fictitious beneficiaries" of scientific projects (Nowotny, 2014, p. 17). This invocation of an unspecified or fictitious 'public good' (as it is framed in relation to medical research participation) obscures the value commitments of science, which should therefore be interrogated in the context of any democratization of science (Irwin, 2014). Such democratization is not just a matter of interrogating or critiquing scientific expertise. As Yaron Ezrahi (2012, p. 133) has observed, "the social authority of science" has long been "an indispensable political resource of the modern liberal democratic state". As a consequence, rejecting science's contribution to solving social problems outright may end in a simultaneous disintegration of democracy itself—as we seem to be witnessing at present. Nevertheless, politics in a functioning democracy should involve "a clash of legitimate democratic political positions" (Mouffe, 2011, p. 30). As a consequence, the value commitments and social effects of scientific research should be open to interrogation in a robust democracy. Science and technology permeate virtually every aspect of life at present, but this does not mean that technoscientific expertise can therefore be the ultimate arbitrator of any and all matters of public concern. Rather, public trust in science requires simultaneous scientific trust in and openness towards the concerns of the public (Bijker, 2017). Rather than to ask about citizens' obligations to participate in medical research, we should therefore oblige medical science to engage with citizens' more-than-scientific concerns around science, health, disease and social rights.

Notes

1. Although these areas of research overlap as much as geographic locations are not isolated. Without engaging in a full discussion of interdisciplinarity in medical research, my case studies show examples of genomics research in epidemiology (Framingham Heart Study) or the increasing relevance of chronic conditions and the so-called epidemiological transition in global health (Million Death Study).
2. Nor is the study sample today representative of the Framingham population, since it has based subsequent cohorts on the initial sample, while the population of Framingham itself has changed and become more ethnically diverse.
3. Not to mention that one study suggests that the paradox is overblown because the quality of European research is not that great to begin with (Rodríguez-Navarro & Narin, 2017)—an argument based on the rather narrow basis of supposed "high impact" publications.
4. I continue to use the term engagement rather than participation to avoid confusion.
5. For a broader critique of the assumption that innovation is a 'panacea' for all social problems and can form a substitute for political debate and decision-making on how to solve societal problems see, e.g., (Pfotenhauer & Jasanoff, 2017; Pfotenhauer & Juhl, 2017).

Bibliography

Aarden, E. (2016). Constitutions of justice in genetic medicine: Distributing diagnostics for familial hypercholesterolemia in three European countries. *Critical Policy Studies, 10*(2), 216–234. https://doi.org/10.1080/19460171.2015.1024704

Aarden, E. (2017a). Making value(s) through social contracts for biomedical population research. In V. Pavone & J. Goven (Eds.), *Bioeconomies: Life, technology and capital in the 21st century* (pp. 161–184). Palgrave Macmillan. https://link.springer.com/chapter/10.1007/978-3-319-55651-2_7

Aarden, E. (2017b). Projecting and producing 'usefulness' of biomedical research infrastructures; or why the Singapore tissue network closed. *Science and Public Policy, 44*(6), 753–762. https://doi.org/10.1093/scipol/scx010

Aarden, E. (2018). Repositioning biological citizenship: State, population and individual risk in the Framingham heart study. *BioSocieties, 13*(2), 494–512. https://doi.org/10.1057/s41292-017-0081-0

Aarden, E. (2019). Decoding the million death study. Ambivalence of producing evidence on mortality in India. *Economic and Political Weekly, 54*(50), 41–48.

Aarden, E. (2021). Human sensing infrastructures and global public health security in India's million death study. In N. Klimburg-Witjes, N. Poechhacker,

E. Aarden, *Producing Citizenship in Medical Research Collections*, Health, Technology and Society, https://doi.org/10.1007/978-981-95-1707-7

& G. Bowker (Eds.), *Sensing in/security. Sensors as international security infrastructures* (pp. 136–162). Manchester: Mattering Press.

Aarden, E. (2023). Infrastructuring European scientific integration: Heterogeneous meanings of the European biobanking infrastructure BBMRI-ERIC. *Social Studies of Science, 53*(4), 572–598. https://doi.org/10.1177/03063127231162629

Aarden, E. (2024). 'Samples are precious': Value formations in the potentialities and practices of biobanking in Singapore. *Science, Technology & Human Values, 49*(3), 500–523. https://doi.org/10.1177/01622439211069129

Aarden, E. (2025). Mapping materials, drawing Europe: Sample and data quality and accessibility in the biobanking infrastructure BBMRI-ERIC. *Big Data & Society, 12*(1), 1–13. https://doi.org/10.1177/20539517241303128

Aarden, E., Van Hoyweghen, I., & Horstman, K. (2011). Constructing access in predictive medicine. Comparing classification for hereditary breast cancer risks in England, Germany and The Netherlands. *Social Science & Medicine, 72*(6), 553–559. https://doi.org/10.1016/j.socscimed.2010.11.033

Aarden, E., Marelli, L., & Blasimme, A. (2021). The translational lag narrative in policy discourse in the United States and the European Union: A comparative study. *Humanities & Social Sciences Communications, 8*, 107. https://doi.org/10.1057/s41599-021-00777-y

Abraham, I. (2006). The contradictory spaces of postcolonial techno-science. *Economic and Political Weekly, 41*, 210–217.

Adams, V. (2013). Evidence-based global public health. Subjects, profits, erasures. In J. Biehl & A. Petryna (Eds.), *When people come first. Critical studies in global health* (pp. 54–90). Princeton: Princeton University Press.

Adams, V. (2016). *Metrics. What counts in global health.* Durham: Duke University Press.

Adjekum, A., Ienca, M., & Vayena, E. (2017). What is trust? Ethics and risk governance in precision medicine and predictive analytics. *OMICS A Journal of Integrative Biology, 21*(12), 704. https://doi.org/10.1089/omi.2017.0156

Akyüz, K., Abadía, M. C., Goisauf, M., Michaela, T., & Mayrhofer. (2024). Unlocking the potential of big data and AI in medicine: Insights from biobanking. *Frontiers in Medicine, 11*, 1336588. https://doi.org/10.3389/fmed.2024.1336588

Amoakoh-Coleman, M., Vieira, D., & Abugri, J. (2023). Ethical considerations for biobanking and use of genomics data in Africa: A narrative review. *BMC Medical Ethics, 24*(1), 108. https://doi.org/10.1186/s12910-023-00985-y

Anand, N., Gupta, A., & Appel, H. (2018). *The promise of infrastructure.* Durham: Duke University Press.

Anderson, B. (2006). *Imagined communities. Reflections on the origins and spread of nationalism*. London: Verso.

Anderson, W. (2009). From subjugated knowledge to conjugated subjects: Science and globalisation, or postcolonial studies of science? *Postcolonial Studies, 12*(4), 289–400. https://doi.org/10.1080/13688790903350641

Anderson, W. (2021). The model crisis, or how to have critical promiscuity in the time of COVID-19. *Social Studies of Science, 51*(2), 167–188. https://doi.org/10.1177/0306312721996053

Ankeny, R., & Leonelli, S. (2015). Valuing data in postgenomic biology. How data donation and curation practices challenge the scientific publication system. In S. Richardson & H. Stevens (Eds.), *Postgenomics. Perspectives on biology after the genome* (pp. 126–149). Durham: Duke University Press.

Annaratone, L., De Palma, G., Bonizzi, G., Sapino, A., Botti, G., Berrino, E., Mannelli, C., et al. (2021). Basic principles of biobanking: From biological samples to precision medicine for patients. *Virchows Archiv, 479*(2), 233–246. https://doi.org/10.1007/s00428-021-03151-0

Appel, H., Anand, N., & Gupta, A. (2018). Introduction. Temporality, politics, and the promise of infrastructure. In N. Anand, A. Gupta, & H. Appel (Eds.), *The promise of infrastructure* (pp. 1–38). Durham: Duke Univeristy Press.

Argudo-Portal, V., & Domènech, M. (2020). The reconfiguration of biobanks in Europe under the BBMRI-ERIC framework: Towards global sharing nodes? *Life Sciences, Society and Policy, 16*(9), 1–15. https://doi.org/10.1186/s40504-020-00105-3

Armstrong, D. (2019). The social life of data points: Antecedents of digital technologies. *Social Studies of Science, 49*(1), 102–117. https://doi.org/10.1177/0306312718821726

Aronowitz, R. (1998). *Making sense of illness: Science, society and disease*. Cambridge: Cambridge University Press.

Asslaber, M., & Zatloukal, K. (2007). Biobanks: Transnational, European and global networks. *Briefings in Functional Genomics and Proteomics, 6*(3), 193–201. https://doi.org/10.1093/bfgp/elm023

Badenoch, A., & Fickers, A. (2010). Introduction Europe materializing? Toward a transnational history of European infrastructures. In A. Badenoch & A. Fickers (Eds.), *Materializing Europe* (pp. 1–23). Basingstoke: Palgrave Macmillan UK. http://link.springer.com/10.1057/9780230292314_1

Baker, M. (2016). 1,500 Scientists lift the lid on reproducibility. *Nature, 533*, 452–454. https://doi.org/10.1038/533452a

Ban, K. C., Pakir, A., & Tong, C. K. (2004). *Imagining Singapore* (2nd ed.). Singapore: Eastern Universities Press.

Barrett, C. D., & Yaffe, M. B. (2020). COVID-19: All the wrong moves in all the wrong places. *Science Signaling, 13*(649), eabe4242. https://doi.org/10.1126/scisignal.abe4242

Barry, A. (2001). *Political machines. Governing a technological society*. London: The Athlone Press.

Barry, A. (2006). Technological zones. *European Journal of Social Theory, 9*(2), 239–253. https://doi.org/10.1177/1368431006063343

Bates, J., Lin, Y., & Goodale, P. (2016). Data journeys: Capturing the socio-material constitution of data objects and flows. *Big Data & Society, 3*, 1–12. https://doi.org/10.1177/2053951716654502

BBMRI-ERIC. (2014). *Work programme 2015*. Graz: BBMRI-ERIC.

BBMRI-ERIC. (2015a). *Biobanks Europe Newsletter 2*. Graz: BBMRI-ERIC.

BBMRI-ERIC. (2015b). *Work programme 2016*. Graz: BBMRI-ERIC.

BBMRI-ERIC. (2016a). *2015 Annual report*. Graz: BBMRI-ERIC.

BBMRI-ERIC. (2016b). *Biobanks Europe 5*. Graz: BBMRI-ERIC.

BBMRI-ERIC. (2016c). *Statutes of the biobanking and biomolecular resources research infrastructures European Research Infrastructure Consortium (BBMRI-ERIC). Rev2*. Graz: BBMRI-ERIC.

BBMRI-ERIC. (2016d). *Work programme 2017*. Graz: BBMRI-ERIC.

BBMRI-ERIC. (2017a). *2016 Annual report*. Graz: BBMRI-ERIC.

BBMRI-ERIC. (2017b). *Biobanks Europe Magazine 6*. Graz: BBMRI-ERIC.

BBMRI-ERIC. (2017c). *Biobanks Europe Magazine 7*. Graz: BBMRI-ERIC.

BBMRI-ERIC. (2018). *BBMRI-ERIC vision paper*. Graz: BBMRI-ERIC.

BBMRI-ERIC. (2019a). *2018 Annual report*. Graz: BBMRI-ERIC.

BBMRI-ERIC. (2019b). *Work programme 2020*. Graz: BBMRI-ERIC.

BBMRI-ERIC. (2020). *2019 Annual report*. Graz: BBMRI-ERIC.

Bell, K. (2017). *Health and other unassailable values. Reconfigurations of health, evidence, and ethics*. London: Routledge.

Beltrami, E. J., Brown, A. C., Salmon, P. J. M., Leffell, D. J., Ko, J. M., & Grant-Kels, J. M. (2022). Artificial intelligence in the detection of skin cancer. *Journal of the American Academy of Dermatology, 87*(6), 1336–1342. https://doi.org/10.1016/j.jaad.2022.08.028

Benjamin, R. (2009). A lab of their own: Genomic sovereignty as postcolonial science policy. *Policy & Society, 28*(4), 341–355. https://doi.org/10.1016/j.polsoc.2009.09.007

Benjamin, R. (2013). *People's science. Bodies and rights on the stem cell frontier*. Stanford: Stanford University Press.

Benner, M. (2018). *The new global politics of science. Knowledge, markets and the state*. Cheltenham: Edward Elgar.

Bhutta, Z. (2006). The million death study in India: Can it help in monitoring the millennium development goals? *PLoS Medicine, 3*(2), e103. https://doi.org/10.1371/journal.pmed.0030103

Biehl, J., & Petryna, A. (2013). Critical global health. In J. Biehl & A. Petryna (Eds.), *When people come first. Critical studies in global health* (pp. 1–20). Princeton: Princeton University Press.

Bijker, W. (1995). *Of bicycles, bakelites and bulbs. Towards a theory of sociotechnical change*. Cambridge: The MIT Press.

Bijker, W. (2017). Constructing worlds: Reflections on science, technology and democracy (and a plea for bold modesty). *Engaging Science, Technology, and Society, 3*, 315–331. https://doi.org/10.17351/ests2017.170

Bijker, W., & Pinch, T. (1987). The social construction of facts and artifacts: Or how the sociology of science and the sociology of technology might benefit each other. In W. Bijker, T. Hughes, & T. Pinch (Eds.), *The social construction of technological systems. New directions in the sociology and history of technology* (pp. 17–50). Cambridge: The MIT Press.

Birbeck, G., Wiysonge, C., Mills, E., Frenk, J., Zhou, X., & Jha, P. (2013). Global health: The importance of evidence-based medicine. *BMC Medicine, 11*, 223. https://doi.org/10.1186/1741-7015-11-223

Birch, K., & Muniesa, F. (Eds.). (2020). *Assetization: Turning things into assets in technoscientific capitalism*. Cambridge: The MIT Press.

Birch, K., & Tyfield, D. (2013). Theorizing the bioeconomy: Biovalue, biocapital, bioeconomics or...What? *Science, Technology & Human Values, 38*(3), 299–327. https://doi.org/10.1177/0162243912442398

Birmingham, K. (2001). Singapore pushes biomedical research. *Nature Medicine, 7*(11), 1169–1170. https://doi.org/10.1038/nm1101-1169

Birn, A. (2009). The stages of international (global) health: Histories of success or successes of history? *Global Public Health: An International Journal for Research, Policy and Practice, 4*(1), 50–68. https://doi.org/10.1080/17441690802017797

Biruk, C. (2012). Seeing like a research project: Producing 'high quality data' in AIDS research in Malawi. *Medical Anthropology: Cross-Cultural Studies in Health and Illness., 31*(4), 347–366. https://doi.org/10.1080/01459740.2011.631960

Biruk, C. (2022). Assembling population data in the field: The labour, technologies, and materialities of quantification. In M. H. Bruun, A. Wahlberg, R. Douglas-Jones, C. Hasse, K. Hoeyer, D. B. Kristensen, & B. R. Winthereik (Eds.), *The Palgrave handbook of the anthropology of technology* (pp. 309–329). Singapore: Springer Nature Singapore. https://doi.org/10.1007/978-981-16-7084-8_16

Bluche, L., Lipphardt, V., & Patel, K. (2009). *Der Europäer – Ein Konstrukt*. Göttingen: Wallstein Verlag.

Blümel, C. (2018). Translational research in the science policy debate: A comparative analysis of documents. *Science & Public Policy*, 45(1), 4-35, https://doi.org/10.1093/scipol/scx034

Borup, M., Brown, N., Konrad, K., & Van Lente, H. (2006). The sociology of expectations in science and technology. *Technology Analysis & Strategic Management, 18*(3/4), 285–298. https://doi.org/10.1080/09537320600777002

Bowker, G., & Star, S. L. (1999). *Sorting things out. Classification and its consequences*. Cambridge: The MIT Press.

boyd, d., & Crawford, K. (2012). Critical questions for big data. *Information, Communication & Society, 15*(5), 662–679. https://doi.org/10.1080/1369118X.2012.678878

Brandt, A. (2007). *The cigarette century. The rise, fall, and deadly persistence of the product that defined America*. New York: Basic Books.

Brown, T., Cueto, M., & Fee, E. (2006). The World Health Organization and the transition from 'international' to 'global' public health. *American Journal of Public Health, 96*(1), 62–72. https://doi.org/10.2105/ajph.2004.050831

Brown, T., Craddock, S., & Ingram, A. (2012). Critical interventions in global health: Governmentality, risk, and assemblage. *Annals of the Association of American Geographers., 102*(5), 1182–1189. https://doi.org/10.1080/00045608.2012.659960

Brunsson, N., & Jacobsson, B. (2002). *A world of standards*. Oxford: Oxford University Press. https://doi.org/10.1093/acprof:oso/9780199256952.001.0001

Bruun Jensen, C., & Morita, A. (2015). Infrastructures as ontological experiments. *Engaging Science, Technology, and Society, 1*, 81–87. https://doi.org/10.1080/00141844.2015.1107607

Burton, D., Saheli, K. K., Paul, K., Samuel, G., & Prainsack, B. (2021). Rethinking value construction in biomedicine and healthcare. *BioSocieties, 17*, 391–414. https://doi.org/10.1057/s41292-020-00220-6

Busby, H., & Martin, P. (2006). Biobanks, national identity and imagined communities: The case of UK biobank. *Science as Culture, 15*(3), 237–251. https://doi.org/10.1080/09505430600890693

Busch, L. (2011). *Standards. Recipes for reality*. Cambridge: The MIT Press.

Butler, D. (2008). Crossing the valley of death. *Nature, 453*, 840–842. https://doi.org/10.1038/453840a

Butler, D. (2010). Verbal autopsy methods questioned. *Nature, 467*, 1015. https://doi.org/10.1038/4671015a

Callon, M., & Latour, B. (1981). Unscrewing the big leviathan: How actors macrostructure reality and sociologists help them to do so. In K. Knorr-Cetina & A. Cicourel (Eds.), *Advances in social theory and methodology: Towards an integration of micro- and macro-sociologies* (pp. 227–303). London: Routledge & Kegan Paul.

Cambrosio, A., Keating, P., Schlich, T., & Weisz, G. (2006). Regulatory objectivity and the generation and management of evidence in medicine. *Social Science & Medicine, 63*, 189–199. https://doi.org/10.1016/j.socscimed.2005.12.007

Cañada, J., Tupasela, A., & Snell, K. (2015). Beyond and within public engagement: A broadened approach to engagement in biobanking. *New Genetics and Society, 34*(4), 355–376. https://doi.org/10.1080/14636778.2015.1105130

Celermajer, D., & McKibbin, P. (2023). Reimagining relationships: Multispecies justice as a frame for the COVID-19 pandemic. *Journal of Bioethical Inquiry, 20*(4), 657–666. https://doi.org/10.1007/s11673-023-10280-5

Chadwick, R., & Strange, H. (2009). Harmonization and standardization in ethics and governance: Conceptual and practical challenges. In H. Widdows & C. Mullen (Eds.), *The governance of genetic information. Who decides?* (pp. 201–213). Cambridge: Cambridge University Press.

Chan, T. W. (2012). The closure of the National Biobank in Singapore. *Asia-Pacific Biotech News Journal, 16*(1), 40–43.

Chan, C., & Liu, E. (2010). The impact of the bioethics advisory committee on the research community in Singapore. In J. Elliott, W. Ho, & S. Lim (Eds.), *Bioethics in Singapore. The ethical microcosm* (pp. 31–49). Singapore: World Scientific.

Chang, A.-L. (2011, June 4). National Biobank to close. *The Straits Times*.

Check Hayden, E. (2010). Human genome at ten: Life is complicated. *Nature, 464*(7289), 664–667. https://doi.org/10.1038/464664a

Chiapetta, M., & Birch, K. (2018). Limits to biocapital. In S. Hilgartner, S. Gibbon, B. Prainsack, & J. Lamoreaux (Eds.), *The Routledge handbook of genomics, health and society* (pp. 63–70). London: Routledge.

Chilvers, J., & Kearnes, M. (2016). Participation in the making. Rethinking public engagement in co-productionist terms. In J. Chilvers & M. Kearnes (Eds.), *Remaking participation. Science, environment and emergent publics* (pp. 31–63). Routledge.

Cho, M. K., Varsava, N., Kraft, S. A., Ashwal, G., Gillespie, K., Magnus, D., Ormond, K. E., Thomas, A., Wilfond, B. S., & Lee, S. S.-J. (2018). Metaphors matter: From biobank to a library of medical information. *Genetics in Medicine, 20*(8), 802–805. https://doi.org/10.1038/gim.2017.204

Chowdhury, J. (2015). National health policy 2015. A narrow focus needed. *Economic & Political Weekly, 50*(9), 25–30.

Choy, T. (2011). *Ecologies of comparison. An ethnography of endangerment in Hong Kong*. Durham: Duke University Press.

Chua, B. H. (2005). Welfare developmentalism in Singapore and Malaysia. In H. J. Kwon (Ed.), *Transforming the developmental welfare state in East Asia* (pp. 98–117). Basingstoke: Palgrave Macmillan.

Clancey, G. (2012). Intelligent Island to biopolis: Smart minds, sick bodies and millennial turns in Singapore. *Science, Technology & Society, 17*(1), 13–35. https://doi.org/10.1177/097172181101700102

Clarke, A. (2005). *Situational analysis. Grounded theory after the postmodern turn*. London: Sage.

Clarke, A., Mamo, L., Fosket, J., Fishman, J., & Shim, J. (2010). *Biomedicalization. Technoscience, health, and illness in the U.S.* Durham: Duke University Press.

Clarke, A., Friese, C., & Washburn, R. (Eds.). (2015). *Situational analysis in practice. Mapping research with grounded theory*. Walnut Creek: Left Coast Press.

Clément, B., Yuille, M., Zaltoukal, K., Wichmann, H.-E., Anton, G., Parodi, B., Kozera, L., et al. (2014). Public biobanks: Calculation and recovery of costs. *Science Translational Medicine, 6*(261), 261fs45. https://doi.org/10.1126/scitranslmed.3010444

Cockerham, W. (2013). *Social causes of health and disease*. Cambridge: Polity Press.

Cohn, B. (1987). The census, social structure and objectification in South Asia. In B. Cohn (Ed.), *An anthropologist among the historians and other essays* (pp. 224–254). Oxford: Oxford University Press.

Cohn, B. (1996). *Colonialism and its forms of knowledge. The British in India*. Princeton:Princeton University Press.

Cohrs, R., Martin, T., Ghahramani, P., Bidaut, L., Higgins, P., & Shahzad, A. (2015). Translational medicine definition by the European Society for Translational Medicine. *New Horizons in Translational Medicine, 2*, 86–88. https://doi.org/10.1016/j.nhtm.2014.12.002

Cole, C., Allen, E., & Feinleib, M. (1974). Section 3. Some characteristics of the Framingham cohort on the first 7 examinations by broad age groups. In *The Framingham study. An epidemiological investigation of cardiovascular disease*. Bethesda: Department of Health, Education, and Welfare, National Institutes of Health.

Collier, S., & Ong, A. (2005). Global assemblages, anthropological problems. In A. Ong & S. Collier (Eds.), *Global assemblages. Technology, politics and ethics as anthropological problems* (pp. 3–21). Malden: Blackwell Publishing.

Collier, S., Mizes, J., & Von Schnitzler, A. (2016). *Preface: Public infrastructures/infrastructural publics*. LIMN. https://limn.press/article/preface-public-infrastructures-infrastructural-publics/

Collins, F. (2011). Reengineering translational science: The time is right. *Science Translational Medicine, 3*(90), 1–6. https://doi.org/10.1126/scitranslmed.3002747

Cool, A. (2016). Detaching data from the state: Biobanking and building big data in Sweden. *BioSocieties, 11*(3), 277–295. https://doi.org/10.1057/biosoc.2015.25

Cool, A. (2022). Peopled by data: Statistical knowledge practices, population-making, and the state. In M. H. Bruun, A. Wahlberg, R. Douglas-Jones, C. Hasse, K. Hoeyer, D. B. Kristensen, & B. R. Winthereik (Eds.), *The Palgrave handbook of the anthropology of technology* (pp. 331–353). Singapore: Springer Nature Singapore. https://doi.org/10.1007/978-981-16-7084-8_17

Cooper, M. (2008). *Life as surplus. Biotechnology and capitalism in the neoliberal era*. Seattle: University of Washington Press.

Cooper, M., & Waldby, C. (2014). *Clinical labor. Tissue donors and research subjects in the global bioeconomy*. Durham: Duke University Press.

Coopmans, C., & Tan, M. (2018). On 'Asian' distinctiveness and race as a variable: The case of ophthalmic epidemiology in Singapore. *Science, Technology & Society, 23*(2), 252–270. https://doi.org/10.1177/0971721818762865

Coopmans, C., Graham, C., & Hamzah, H. (2012). The lab, the clinic, and the image: Working on translational research in Singapore's eye care realm. *Science, Technology & Society, 17*(1), 57–77. https://doi.org/10.1177/097172181101700104

Cooter, R. (2008). Biocitizenship. *The Lancet, 372*, 1752. https://doi.org/10.1016/s0140-6736(08)61719-5

Cramer, K., Hallonsten, O., Bolliger, I., & Griffiths, A. (2020). Big science and research infrastructures in Europe: History and current trends. In K. Cramer & O. Hallonsten (Eds.), *Big science and research infrastructures in Europe* (pp. 1–26). Cheltenham: Edward Elgar.

Crane, J. (2010). Unequal 'partners'. AIDS, academia and the rise of global health. *Behemoth: A Journal of Civilization, 3*, 78–97. https://doi.org/10.1524/behe.2010.0021

Curtis, B. (2002). *The politics of population: State formation, statistics, and the census of Canada, 1840–1875*. Toronto: University of Toronto Press.

Cyranoski, D. (2001). Building a biopolis. *Nature, 412*, 370–371. https://doi.org/10.1038/35086696

da Silva Torres, M. K., Bichara, C. D. A., de Almeida, M. N. D. S., Vallinoto, M. C., Queiroz, M. A. F., Vallinoto, I. M. V. C., Dos Santos, E. J. M., de Carvalho, C. A. M., & Vallinoto, A. C. R. (2022). The complexity of SARS-CoV-2 infection and the COVID-19 pandemic. *Frontiers in Microbiology, 13*, 789882. https://doi.org/10.3389/fmicb.2022.789882

Daemmrich, A. (2004). *Pharmacopolitics. Drug regulation in the United States and Germany*. Chapel Hill: University of North Carolina Press.

Dandara, C., Huzair, F., Borda-Rodriguez, A., Chirikure, S., Okpechi, I., Warnich, L., & Masimirembwa, C. (2014). H3Africa and the African life sciences ecosystem: Building sustainable innovation. *OMICS: A Journal of Integrative Biology, 18*(12), 733–739. https://doi.org/10.1089/omi.2014.0145

Das, V., & Poole, D. (2004). State and its margins: Comparative ethnographies. In V. Das & D. Poole (Eds.), *Anthropology in the margins of the state* (pp. 3–33). Santa Fe: School of American Research Press.

Davies, G., Frow, E., & Leonelli, S. (2013). Bigger, faster, better? Rhetorics and practices of large-scale research in contemporary bioscience. *BioSocieties, 8*(4), 386–396. https://doi.org/10.1057/biosoc.2013.26

Davis, R. L., & Khoury, M. J. (2007). The emergence of biobanks: Practical design considerations for large population-based studies of gene-environment interactions. *Community Genetics, 10*(3), 181–185. https://doi.org/10.1159/000101760

Dawber, T. R. (1980). *The Framingham study*. Cambridge: Harvard University Press.

Dawber, T. R., & Kannel, W. B. (1966). The Framingham study an epidemiological approach to coronary heart disease. *Circulation, 34*(4), 553–555. https://doi.org/10.1161/01.cir.34.4.553

de Vries, J., Munung, S. N., Matimba, A., McCurdy, S., Oukem-Boyer, O. O. M., Staunton, C., Yakubu, A., Tindana, P., & the H3Africa Consortium. (2017). Regulation of genomic and biobanking research in Africa: A content analysis of ethics guidelines, policies and procedures from 22 African countries. *BMC Medical Ethics, 18*(1), 8. https://doi.org/10.1186/s12910-016-0165-6

Deaton, A. (2013). *The great escape: Health, wealth, and the origins of inequality*. Princeton: Princeton University Press.
Delanty, G. (2002). Models of European identity: Reconciling universalism and particularism. *Perspectives on European Politics and Society, 3*(3), 345–359. https://doi.org/10.1080/15705850208438841
DelVecchio Good, M. (2007). The medical imaginary and the biotechnical embrace: Subjective experiences of clinical scientists and patients. In J. Biehl, B. Good, & A. Kleinman (Eds.), *Subjectivity. Ethnographic investigations* (pp. 362–380). Berkeley:University of California Press.
Desai, N., Aleksandrowicz, L., Miasnikof, P., Lu, Y., Leitao, J., Byass, P., Tollman, S., et al. (2014). Performance of four computer-coded verbal autopsy methods for cause of death assignment compared with physician coding on 24,000 deaths in Low- and middle-income countries. *BMC Medicine, 12*(20), 1–8. https://doi.org/10.1186/1741-7015-12-20
Deville, J., Guggenheim, M., & Hrdlickova, Z. (2016). Introduction: The practices and infrastructures of comparison. In J. Deville, M. Guggenheim, & Z. Hrdlickova (Eds.), *Practising comparison: Logics, relations, collaborations* (pp. 17–41). Manchester: Mattering Press.
Dhingra, N., Jha, P., Sharma, V., Cohen, A., Jotkar, R., Rodriguez, P., Bassani, D., et al. (2010). Adult and child malaria mortality in India: A nationally representative mortality survey. *The Lancet, 376*, 1768–1774. https://doi.org/10.1016/S0140-6736(10)60831-8
Dingwall, R., Hoffman, L. M., & Staniland, K. (2013). Introduction: Why a sociology of pandemics? *Sociology of Health & Illness, 35*(2), 167–173. https://doi.org/10.1111/1467-9566.12019
Doing, P. (2008). Give me a laboratory and I Will raise a discipline: The past, present, and future politics of laboratory studies in STS. In E. Hackett, O. Amsterdamska, M. Lynch, & J. Wajcman (Eds.), *The handbook of science and technology studies* (3rd ed., pp. 279–296). Cambridge: The MIT Press.
Doucet, M., Yuille, M., Georghiu, L., & Dagher, G. (2017). Biobank sustainability: Current status and future prospects. *Journal of Biorepository Science for Applied Medicine, 5*, 1–7. https://doi.org/10.2147/BSAM.S100899
Drèze, J., & Sen, A. (2013). *An uncertain glory. India and its contradictions*. Princeton: Princeton University Press.
Duclos Lindstrøm, M., & Kropp, K. (2017). Understanding the infrastructure of European research infrastructures – The case of the European Social Survey (ESS-ERIC). *Science and Public Policy, 44*(6), 855–864. https://doi.org/10.1093/scipol/scx018

Dunn, E. (2005). Standards and person-making in east Central Europe. In A. Ong & S. Collier (Eds.), *Global assemblages. Technology, politics and ethics as anthropological problems* (pp. 173–193). Malden: Blackwell Publishing.

Dussauge, I., Helgesson, C.-F., & Lee, F. (2015a). *Value practices in the life sciences & medicine*. Oxford: Oxford University Press.

Dussauge, I., Helgesson, C.-F., & Lee, F. (2015b). Valuography. Studying the making of values. In I. Dussauge, C.-F. Helgesson, & F. Lee (Eds.), *Value practices in the life sciences & medicine* (pp. 267–285). Oxford: Oxford University Press.

Dussauge, I., Helgesson, C.-F., Lee, F., & Woolgar, S. (2015c). On the omnipresence, diversity, and elusiveness of values in the life sciences and medicine. In I. Dussauge, C.-F. Helgesson, & F. Lee (Eds.), *Value practices in the life sciences & medicine* (pp. 1–28). Oxford University Press.

Dwyer, J., & Feinleib, M. (1992). Introduction to statistical methods for longitudinal observation. In J. Dwyer, M. Feinleib, P. Lippert, & H. Hoffmeister (Eds.), *Statistical models for longitudinal studies of health* (pp. 3–48). Oxford University Press.

Economic and Political Weekly. (2015). Editorial. Long on eloquence, short on detail. *Economic & Political Weekly, 50*(4), 8–9.

Epstein, F. (1992). Contribution of epidemiology to understanding coronary heart disease. In M. Marmot & P. Elliott (Eds.), *Coronary heart disease epidemiology. From aetiology to public health* (pp. 20–32). Oxford University Press.

Escobar, A. (2011). *Encountering development. The making and unmaking of the third world*. Princeton University Press.

Espeland, W., & Stevens, M. (2008). A sociology of quantification. *European Journal of Sociology, 49*(3), 401–436. https://doi.org/10.1017/S0003975609000150

Etzkowitz, H. (2008). *The triple helix: Industry, university, and government in innovation*. Routledge.

Eubanks, V. (2017). *Automating inequality. How high-tech tools profile, police, and punish the poor*. St. Martin's Press.

European Strategy Forum on Research Infrastructures. (2006). *Roadmap for European research infrastructure: Report of the physical sciences and engineering roadmap working group*. https://ec.europa.eu/research/infrastructures/pdf/esfri/esfri_roadmap/roadmap_2006/pse-report-roadmap-wg-2006_en.pdf#view=fit&pagemode=none

Ezrahi, Y. (2012). *Imagined democracies: Necessary political fictions*. Cambridge University Press.

Faulks, K. (2000). *Citizenship*. Routledge.

Feinleib, M., Kannel, W. B., Castelli, W., & McNamara, P. (1968). Section 8. Two-year incidence by exam interval by age at exam 1 and sex. In *The Framingham study. An epidemiological investigation of cardiovascular disease*. US Department of Health, Education and Welfare, Naional Institutes of Health.

Feinleib, M., Kannel, W. B., Garison, R., McNamara, P., & Castelli, W. (1975). The Framingham offspring study. Design and preliminary data. *Preventive Medicine, 4*, 518–525. https://doi.org/10.1016/0091-7435(75)90037-7

Felt, U., Fochler, M., & Winkler, P. (2010). Coming to terms with biomedical technologies in different technopolitical cultures: A comparative analysis of focus groups on organ transplantation and genetic testing in Austria, France, and the Netherlands. *Science, Technology & Human Values, 35*(4), 525–553. https://doi.org/10.1177/0162243909345839

Felt, U., Felder, K., & Penkler, M. (2017). How differences matter: Tracing diversity practices in obesity treatment and health promotion. *Sociology of Health & Illness, 39*(1), 127–142. https://doi.org/10.1111/1467-9566.12446

Fernandez Lynch, H., & Joffe, S. (2017, April 21). Science needs your cells. *The New York Times*.

Fischer, M. (2007). Four genealogies for a recombinant anthropology of science and technology. *Cultural Anthropology, 22*(4), 539–613. https://doi.org/10.1525/can.2007.22.4.539

Fischer, M. (2013). Biopolis: Asian science in the global circuitry. *Science, Technology & Society, 18*(3), 379–404. https://doi.org/10.1177/0971721813498500

Fischer, M. (2018). A tale of two genome institutes: Qualitative networks, charismatic voice, and R&D strategies – Juxtaposing GIS biopolis and BGI. *Science, Technology & Society, 23*(2), 271–288. https://doi.org/10.1177/0971721818762876

Fiske, A., Degelsegger-Márquez, A., Marsteurer, B., & Prainsack, B. (2022). Value-creation in the health data domain: A typology of what health data help us do. *BioSocieties*. https://doi.org/10.1057/s41292-022-00276-6

Flint, J. (2013). GWAS. *Current Biology, 23*(7), R265–R266. https://doi.org/10.1016/j.cub.2013.01.040

Fobelets, G., & Nys, H. (2009). Evolution in research biobanks and its legal consequences. In K. Dierickx & P. Borry (Eds.), *New challenges for biobanks: Ethics, law and governance* (pp. 19–29). Intersentia.

Fortun, M. (2008). *Promising genomics. Iceland and deCODE genetics in a world of speculation*. University of California Press.

Foucault, M. (2007). *Security, territory, population. Lectures at the college de France 1977–1978*. Picador.

Foucault, M. (2013). Right of death and power over life. In T. Campbell & A. Sitze (Eds.), *Biopolitics: A reader* (pp. 41–60). Duke University Press.

Funtowicz, S. O., & Ravetz, J. R. (1993). Science for the post-normal age. *Futures, 25*(7), 739–755. https://doi.org/10.1016/0016-3287(93)90022-L

Gardner, J., & Webster, A. (2016). The social management of biomedical novelty: Facilitating translation in regenerative medicine. *Social Science & Medicine, 156*, 90–97. https://doi.org/10.1016/j.socscimed.2016.03.025

Gaskell, G., Gottweis, H., Starkbaum, J., Gerber, M., Broerse, J., Gottweis, U., Hobbs, A., et al. (2013). Publics and biobanks: Pan-European diversity and the challenge of responsible innovation. *European Journal of Human Genetics, 21*(1), 14–20. https://doi.org/10.1038/ejhg.2012.104

Gaudillière, J.-P., & Gasnier, C. (2020). From Washington, DC to Washington State: The global burden of diseases data basis and the political economy of global health. In S. Leonelli & N. Tempini (Eds.), *Data journeys in the sciences* (pp. 351–369). Springer

Gehlbach, S. (2005). Searching America's heart: The Framingham study. In *American plagues: Lessons from our battles with disease*. McGraw-Hill.

Gelfert, A. (2013). Before biopolis: Representations of the biotechnology discourse in Singapore. *East Asian Science, Technology, and Society: An International Journal, 7*(2), 103–123. https://doi.org/10.1215/18752160-2075527

Gibbons, M. (1999). Science's new social contract with society. *Nature, 402*(Suppl 2), C81–C84. https://doi.org/10.1038/35011576

Gibbons, M., Limoges, C., Nowotny, H., Schwartzman, S., Scott, P., & Trow, M. (1994). *The new production of knowledge: The dynamics of science and research in contemporary societies*. Sage.

Gieryn, T. (1995). Boundaries of science. In S. Jasanoff, G. Markle, J. Petersen, & T. Pinch (Eds.), *The handbook of science and technology studies* (pp. 393–443). SAGE.

Gieryn, T. (1999). *Cultural boundaries of science. Credibility on the line*. University of Chicago Press.

Gille, F., Vayena, E., & Blasimme, A. (2020). Future-proofing biobanks' governance. *European Journal of Human Genetics, 28*(8), 989–996. https://doi.org/10.1038/s41431-020-0646-4

Giroux, E. (2013). The Framingham study and the constitution of a restrictive concept of risk factor. *Social History of Medicine, 26*(1), 94–112. https://doi.org/10.1093/shm/hks051

Global Health Watch. (2011). *Global Health Watch 3: An alternative world health report*. Zed Books.

Goisauf, M., & Durnovà, A. (2019). From engaging publics to engaging knowledges: Enacting 'appropriateness' in the Austrian biobank infrastructure. *Public Understanding of Science, 28*(3), 275–289. https://doi.org/10.1177/0963662518806451

Gordon, T. (1968). Section 2. Follow up to the eighth examination. In *The Framingham study. An epidemiological investigation of cardiovascular disease*. US Department of Health, Education and Welfare, National Institutes of Health.

Gordon, T., & Kannel, W. B. (1968). Section 1. Introduction and general background. In *The Framingham study. An epidemiological investigation of cardiovascular disease*. Department of Health, Education and Welfare, National Institutes of Health.

Gottweis, H., & Lauss, G. (2010). Biobank governance in the post-genomic age. *Personalized Medicine, 7*(2), 187–195. https://doi.org/10.2217/pme.10.4

Gottweis, H., & Lauss, G. (2011). Biobank governance: Heterogeneous modes of ordering and democratization. *Journal of Community Genetics, 3*(2), 61–72. https://doi.org/10.1007/s12687-011-0070-0

Gottweis, H., & Petersen, A. (2008). *Biobanks. Governance in comparative perspective*. Routledge.

Gottweis, H., Salter, B., & Waldby, C. (2009). *The global politics of human embryonic stem cell science. Regenerative medicine in transition*. Palgrave Macmillan.

Gottweis, H., Chen, H., & Starkbaum, J. (2011). Biobanks and the phantom public. *Human Genetics, 130*, 433–440. https://doi.org/10.1007/s00439-011-1065-y

Goven, J., & Pavone, V. (2015). The bioeconomy as political project: A Polanyian analysis. *Science, Technology & Human Values, 40*(3), 302–337. https://doi.org/10.1177/0162243914552133

Govindaraju, D. R., Adrienne Cupples, L., Kannel, W. B., O'Donnell, C. J., Atwood, L. D., D'Agostino, R. B., Fox, C. S., et al. (2008). Chapter 2: Genetics of the Framingham heart study population. *Advances in Genetics, 62*, 33–65. https://doi.org/10.1016/s0065-2660(08)00602-0

Grande, D., Mitra, N., Shah, A., Wan, F., & Asch, D. (2014). The importance of purpose: Moving beyond consent in the societal use of personal health information. *Annals of Internal Medicine, 161*, 855–862. https://doi.org/10.7326/m14-1118

Greenberg, H. (2010). The global impact of the Framingham heart study. *Progress in Cardiovascular Diseases, 53*(1), 1–2. https://doi.org/10.1016/j.pcad.2010.05.003

Greene, J. (2007). *Prescribing by numbers. Drugs and the definition of disease.* Johns Hopkins Press.

Greenhalgh, T., Sivan, M., Perlowski, A., & Nikolich, J. Ž. (2024). Long COVID: A clinical update. *The Lancet, 404*(10453), 707–724. https://doi.org/10.1016/S0140-6736(24)01136-X

Gromme, F., & Ruppert, E. (2019). Population geometries of Europe: The topologies of data cubes and grids. *Science, Technology, & Human Values, 45*(2), 235–261. https://doi.org/10.1177/0162243919835302

Guston, D. (2000). *Between politics and science. Assuring the integrity and productivity of research.* Cambridge University Press.

Hacking, I. (2006). Genetics, biosocial groups & the future of identity. *Daedalus, 135*(4), 81–95.

Hallonsten, O. (2012). Continuity and change in the politics of European scientific collaboration. *Journal of Contemporary European Research, 8*(3), 300–319. https://doi.org/10.30950/jcer.v8i3.366

Hallonsten, O. (2020). Research infrastructures in Europe: The hype and the field. *European Review, 28*(4), 617–635. https://doi.org/10.1017/S1062798720000095

Harambam, J. (2020). The corona truth wars: Where have all the STS'ers gone when we need them most? *Science & Technology Studies, 33*(4), 60–67. https://doi.org/10.23987/sts.99550

Harambam, J. (2023). Distrusting consensus: How a uniform corona pandemic narrative fostered suspicion and conspiracy theories. *Journal of Digital Social Research, 5*(3), 109–139. https://doi.org/10.33621/jdsr.v5i3.143

Haraway, D. (1991). Situated knowledges. The science question in feminism and the privilege of partial perspective. In *Simians, cyborgs, and women. The reinvention of nature* (pp. 183–202). Free Association Books.

Harding, S. (2006). *Science and social inequality. Feminist and postcolonial issues.* University of Illinois Press.

Harding, S. (2009). Postcolonial and feminist philosophies of science and technology: Convergence and dissonances. *Postcolonial Studies, 12*(4), 401–421. https://doi.org/10.1080/13688790903350658

Hasseltine, W. (2013). *Affordable excellence. The Singapore healthcare story.* Brookings Institution Press.

Heater, D. (2004). *A brief history of citizenship.* New York University Press.

Heath, D., Rapp, R., & Taussig, K. (2008). Genetic citizenship. In D. Nugent & J. Vincent (Eds.), *A companion to the anthropology of politics* (pp. 152–167). Wiley-Blackwell.

Hertzman, C., & Siddiqi, A. (2009). Population health and the dynamics of collective development. In P. A. Hall & M. Lamont (Eds.), *Successful societies: How institutions and culture affect health* (pp. 23–52). Cambridge University Press. https://doi.org/10.1017/CBO9780511816192.003

Hessels, L., & Van Lente, H. (2008). Re-thinking new knowledge production: A literature review and a research agenda. *Research Policy, 37*, 740–760. https://doi.org/10.1016/j.respol.2008.01.008

Hessels, L., Van Lente, H., & Smits, R. (2009). In search of relevance: The changing contract between science and society. *Science and Public Policy, 36*(5), 387–401. https://doi.org/10.3152/030234209X442034

Hewitt, R., & Hainaut, P. (2011). Biobanking in a fast moving world: An international perspective. *JNCI Monographs, 2011*(42), 50–51. https://doi.org/10.1093/jncimonographs/lgr005

Hilgartner, S. (2017). *Reordering life: Knowledge and control in the genomics revolution*. The MIT Press.

Ho, W. C., & Lim, S. (2010). The coming of bioethics to Singapore. In J. Elliott, W. C. Ho, & S. Lim (Eds.), *Bioethics in Singapore. The ethical microcosm* (pp. 1–29). World Scientific.

Hoeyer, K. (2023). *Data paradoxes. The politics of intensified data sourcing in contemporary healthcare*. The MIT Press.

Holden, K., & Demeritt, D. (2008). Democratising science? The politics of promoting biomedicine in Singapore's developmental state. *Environment and Planning D: Society and Space, 26*, 68–86. https://doi.org/10.1068/d461t

Hurlbut, J. B., Metzler, I., Marelli, L., & Jasanoff, S. (2020). Bioconstitutional imaginaries and the comparative politics of genetic self-knowledge. *Science, Technology, & Human Values, 45*(6), 1087–1118. https://doi.org/10.1177/0162243920921246

Iliadis, A., & Russo, F. (2016). Critical data studies: An introduction. *Big Data & Society, 3*(2), 2053951716674238. https://doi.org/10.1177/2053951716674238

Illich, I. (1975). *Medical nemesis. The expropriation of health*. Calder & Boyars.

Irwin, A. (2014). From deficit to democracy (re-visited). *Public Understanding of Science, 23*(1), 71–76.

Irwin, A. (2015). Science, public engagement with. In *International encyclopaedia of the social & behavioral sciences* (Vol. 21, 2nd ed., pp. 255–260). Centrum Press. https://doi.org/10.1016/B978-0-08-097086-8.85055-2

Jackson, S., & Barbrow, S. (2013). Infrastructure and vocation: Field, calling and computation in ecology. https://doi.org/10.1145/2470654.2481397

Jackson, S., Edwards, P., Bowker, G., & Knobel, C. (2007). Understanding infrastructure: History, heuristics, and cyberinfrastructure policy. *First Monday, 12*(6). https://doi.org/10.5210/fm.v12i6.1904

Jaquish, C. E. (2007). The Framingham heart study, on its way to becoming the gold standard for cardiovascular genetic epidemiology? *BMC Medical Genetics, 8*(1), 63–65. https://doi.org/10.1186/1471-2350-8-63

Jasanoff, S. (2004). *States of knowledge. The co-production of science and social order*. Routledge.

Jasanoff, S. (2005). *Designs on nature. Science and democracy in Europe and the United States*. Princeton University Press.

Jasanoff, S. (Ed.). (2011). *Reframing rights: Bioconstitutionalism in the genetic age*. The MIT Press.

Jasanoff, S. (2020). Pathologies of liberty. Public health sovereignty and the political subject in the COVID-19 crisis. *Cahiers Droit, Sciences & Technologies, 11*, 125–149. https://doi.org/10.4000/cdst.2982

Jasanoff, S., & Kim, S.-h. (2009). Containing the atom: Sociotechnical imaginaries and nuclear power in the United States and South Korea. *Minerva, 47*(2), 119–146. https://doi.org/10.1007/s11024-009-9124-4

Jasanoff, S., & Kim, S.-h. (2015). *Dreamscapes of modernity. Sociotechnical imaginaries and the fabrication of power*. University of Chicago Press.

Jasanoff, S., Hilgartner, S., Hurlbut, B., Özgöde, O., & Rayzberg, M. (2021, January 12). *Comparative COVID response: Crisis, knowledge, politics interim report*. https://compcore.cornell.edu/wp-content/uploads/2021/03/Comparative-Covid-Response_Crisis-Knowledge-Politics_Interim-Report.pdf

Jauho, M., & Helén, I. (2023). Citizenship by vitality: Rethinking the concept of health citizenship. *Distinktion: Journal of Social Theory, 24*(3), 467–487. https://doi.org/10.1080/1600910X.2022.2057561

Jha, P. (2012). Counting the dead is one of the world's best investments to reduce premature mortality. *Hypothesis, 10*(1), e3. https://doi.org/10.5779/hypothesis.v10i1.211

Jha, P. (2014). Reliable direct measurement of causes of death in low- and middle-income countries. *BMC Medicine, 12*(19), 1–10. https://doi.org/10.1186/1741-7015-12-19

Jha, P., & Laxminarayan, R. (2009). *Choosing health. An entitlement for all Indians*. Center for Global Health Research.

Jha, P., Gajalakshmi, V., Gupta, P., Kumar, R., Mony, P., Dhingra, N., Peto, R., & RGI-CGHR Prospective Study Collaborators. (2006). Prospective study of 1 million deaths in India: Rationale, design and validation results. *PLoS Medicine, 3*(2), e18. https://doi.org/10.1371/journal.pmed.0030018

Jogalekar, A. (2012). The perils of translational research. *Scientific American.*

Johnson, J., Happe, K. E., & Levina, M. (2018). Introduction. In K. E. Happe, J. Johnson, & M. Levina (Eds.), *Biocitizenship: The politics of bodies, governance, and power* (pp. 1–18). New York University Press. https://doi.org/10.18574/nyu/9781479845194.003.0001

Jutel, A. (2011). Classification, disease, and diagnosis. *Perspectives in Biology and Medicine, 54*(2), 189–205. https://doi.org/10.1353/pbm.2011.0015

Kaiser, J. (2002). Population databases boom, from Iceland to the U.S. *Science, 298*, 1158–1161. https://doi.org/10.1126/science.298.5596.1158

Kaiser, W., & Schot, J. (2014). *Writing the rules for Europe. Experts, cartels and international organizations.* Palgrave Macmillan.

Kannel, W. B. (1987). New perspectives on cardiovascular risk factors. *American Heart Journal, 114*(1), 213–219. https://doi.org/10.1016/0002-8703(87)90964-1

Kannel, W. B., & Wilson, P. (2007). Risk factors for cardiovascular disease and the Framingham study equation. In A. Gotto & P. Toth (Eds.), *Comprehensive management of high risk cardiovascular patients* (pp. 1–18). Informa Healthcare.

Kannel, W. B., Dawber, T. R., Kagan, A., Revotskie, N., & Stokes, J. (1961). Factors of risk in the development of coronary heart disease – Six year follow-up experience. *Annals of Internal Medicine, 55*(1), 33–50. https://doi.org/10.7326/0003-4819-55-1-33

Kannel, W. B., McGee, D., & Gordon, T. (1976). A general cardiovascular risk profile: The Framingham study. *The American Journal of Cardiology, 38*, 46–51. https://doi.org/10.1016/0002-9149(76)90061-8

Kannel, W. B., Manning Feinleib, P., McNamara, R. G., & Castelli, W. (1979). An investigation of coronary heart disease in families. The Framingham offspring study. *American Journal of Epidemiology, 110*(3), 281–290. https://doi.org/10.1093/oxfordjournals.aje.a112813

Karasti, H., & Blomberg, J. (2018). Studying infrastructuring ethnographically. *Computer Supported Cooperative Work (CSCW), 27*(2), 233–265. https://doi.org/10.1007/s10606-017-9296-7

Kaye, J. (2009). Biobanking networks – What are the governance challenges? In J. Kaye & M. Stranger (Eds.), *Principles and practices in biobank governance* (pp. 201–213). Ashgate.

Kaye, J., & Stranger, M. (2009). *Principles and practice in biobank governance*. Ashgate.

Keating, P., & Cambrosio, A. (2003). *Biomedical platforms. Realigning the normal and the pathological in late twentieth century medicine*. The MIT Press.

Keating, P., Cambrosio, A., & Nelson, N. (2016). 'Triple negative breast cancer': Translational research and the (re)assembling of diseases in post-genomic medicine. *Studies in History and Philosophy of Biological and Biomedical Sciences, 59*(1), 20–34. https://doi.org/10.1016/j.shpsc.2016.05.003

Keller, E. F. (2000). *The century of the gene*. Harvard University Press.

Kerr, A. (2004). *Genetics and society. A sociology of disease*. Routledge.

Kim, S.-h. (2013). The politics of human embryonic stem cell research in South Korea: Contesting national sociotechnical imaginaries. *Science as Culture, 23*(3), 293–319. https://doi.org/10.1080/09505431.2013.860095

Kinkorová, J. (2016). Biobanks in the era of personalized medicine: Objectives, challenges, and innovation. *EPMA Journal, 7*(4), 1–12. https://doi.org/10.1186/s13167-016-0053-7

Kitchin, R. (2014a). Big data, new epistemologies and paradigm shifts. *Big Data & Society, 1*, 1–12. https://doi.org/10.1177/2053951714528481

Kitchin, R. (2014b). *The data revolution: Big data, open data, data infrastructures and their consequences*. SAGE.

Kivisto, P., & Faist, T. (2007). *Citizenship: Discourse, theory and transnational prospects*. Wiley-Blackwell.

Knoppers, B. M. (2005). Of genomics and public health: Building public 'goods'? *CMAJ, 173*(10), 1185–1186. https://doi.org/10.1503/cmaj.050325

Knoppers, B. M., & Abdul-Rahman, M.'n. H. (2008). Biobanks in the literature. In B. Elger, N. Biller-Adorno, A. Mauron, & A. Capron (Eds.), *Ethical issues in governing biobanks. Global perspectives* (pp. 13–22). Ashgate.

Knoppers, B. M., & Abdul-Rahman, M.'n. H. (2009). Health privacy in genetic research: Populations and persons. *Politics and the Life Sciences, 28*(2), 99–101. https://doi.org/10.2990/28_2_99

Knoppers, B. M., & Chadwick, R. (2005). Human genetic research: Emerging trends in ethics. *Nature Reviews Genetics, 6*, 75–79. https://doi.org/10.1038/nrg1505

Knoppers, B. M., & Hudson, T. J. (2011). The art and science of biobanking. *Human Genetics, 130*(3), 329–332. https://doi.org/10.1007/s00439-011-1067-9

Knoppers, B. M., Abdul-Rahman, M.'n. H., & Bédard, K. (2007). Genomic databases and international collaboration. *King's Law Journal, 18*(2), 291–311. https://doi.org/10.1080/09615768.2007.11427678

Knorr-Cetina, K. (1983). The ethnographic study of scientific work: Towards a constructivist interpretation. In K. Knorr-Cetina & M. Mulkay (Eds.), *Science observed: Perspectives on the social study of science* (pp. 115–140). Sage.

Knorr-Cetina, K. (1999). *Epistemic cultures. How the sciences make knowledge.* Harvard University Press.

Knox, H. (2017). Affective infrastructures and the political imagination. *Public Culture, 29*(2), 363–384. https://doi.org/10.1215/08992363-3749105

Koch, T. (2017). *Cartographies of disease: Maps, mapping, and medicine, new* (Expanded edition). Esri Press.

Kohli-Laven, N., Bourret, P., Keating, P., & Cambrosio, A. (2011). Cancer clinical trials in the era of genomic signatures: Biomedical innovation, clinical utility, and regulatory-scientific hybrids. *Social Studies of Science, 41*(4), 487–513. https://doi.org/10.1177/0306312711398741

Kothari, M., & Mehta, L. (1988). Violence in modern medicine. In A. Nandy (Ed.), *Science, hegemony and violence. A requiem for modernity* (pp. 167–210). The United Nations University.

Kowal, E. (2022). Structuring race into the machine: The spoiled promise of postgenomic sequencing technologies. In M. H. Bruun, A. Wahlberg, R. Douglas-Jones, C. Hasse, K. Hoeyer, D. B. Kristensen, & B. R. Winthereik (Eds.), *The Palgrave handbook of the anthropology of technology* (pp. 165–182). Springer Nature Singapore. https://doi.org/10.1007/978-981-16-7084-8_8

Krieger, N. (2012). Who and what is a 'population'? Historical debates, current controversies, and implications for understanding 'population health' and rectifying health inequalities. *The Milbank Quarterly, 90*(4), 634–681. https://doi.org/10.1111/j.1468-0009.2012.00678.x

Kumar, D. (2001). *Disease and medicine in India. A historical overview.* Tulika Books.

Kuo, W. (2012). Transforming states in the era of global pharmaceuticals. Visioning clinical research in Japan, Taiwan, and Singapore. In K. Sunder Rajan (Ed.), *Lively capital. Biotechnologies, ethics, and governance in global markets* (pp. 279–305). Duke University Press.

Lablans, M., Kadioglu, D., Mate, S., Leb, I., Prokosch, H.-U., & Ückert, F. (2016). Strategien Zur Vernetzung von Biobanken. *Bundesgesundheitsblatt – Gesundheitsforschung – Gesundheitsschutz, 59*(3), 373–378. https://doi.org/10.1007/s00103-015-2299-y

Langhof, H., Kahrass, H., Sievers, S., & Strech, D. (2017). Access policies in biobank research: What criteria do they include and how publicly available are they? A cross-sectional study. *European Journal of Human Genetics, 25*, 293–300. https://pubmed.ncbi.nlm.nih.gov/28000694/

Larkin, B. (2013). The politics and poetics of infrastructure. *Annual Review of Anthropology, 42*, 327–343. https://doi.org/10.1146/annurev-anthro-092412-155522

Larkin, B. (2018). Promising forms. The political aesthetics of infrastructure. In N. Anand, A. Gupta, & H. Appel (Eds.), *The promise of infrastructure* (pp. 175–202). Duke University Press.

Laruffa, F. (2022). Toward a post-neoliberal social citizenship? *Constellations, 29*(3), 375–392. https://doi.org/10.1111/1467-8675.12599

Latour, B. (1983). Give me a laboratory and I will raise the world. In K. Knorr-Cetina & M. Mulkay (Eds.), *Science observed* (pp. 141–170). Sage.

Latour, B. (1987). *Science in action. How to follow scientists and engineers through society*. Harvard University Press.

Latour, B. (1999). *Pandora's hope. Essays on the reality of science studies*. Harvard University Press.

Latour, B. (2004). Why has critique run out of steam? From matters of fact to matters of concern. *Critical Inquiry, 30*(2), 225–248. https://doi.org/10.1086/421123

Latour, B., & Woolgar, S. (1986). *Laboratory life. The construction of scientific facts*. Princeton University Press.

Lauss, G. (2009). Orchestrating 'the end of the beginning'. A political science perspective on transnational biobank infrastructures in Europe. In K. Dierickx & P. Borry (Eds.), *New challenges for biobanks: Ethics, law and governance* (pp. 249–267). Intersentia.

Law, J. (2004). *After method. Mess in social science research*. Routledge.

Law, J. (2009). Actor network theory and material semiotics. In B. S. Turner (Ed.), *The new Blackwell companion to social theory* (pp. 143–158). Blackwell Publishing.

Lee, S. A. (2007). *Singapore from place to nation*. Prentice Hall.

Lee, E. (2008). *Singapore. The unexpected nation*. ISEAS Publishing.

Leitao, J., Desai, N., Aleksandrowicz, L., Byass, P., Miasnikof, P., Tollman, S., Alam, D., et al. (2014). Comparison of physician-certified verbal autopsy with computer-coded verbal autopsy for cause of death assignment in hospitalized patients in Low- and middle-income countries: Systematic review. *BMC Medicine, 12*(22), 1–9. https://doi.org/10.1186/1741-7015-12-22

Lemke, T. (2007). *Biopolitik. Zur Einführung*. Junius Verlag.

Leonelli, S. (2012). Introduction: Making sense of data-driven research in the biological and biomedical sciences. *Studies in History and Philosophy of Science Part C: Studies in History and Philosophy of Biological and Biomedical Sciences, 43*(1), 1–3. https://doi.org/10.1016/j.shpsc.2011.10.001

Leonelli, S. (2013). Global data for local science: Assessing the scale of data infrastructures in biological and biomedical researchers. *BioSocieties, 8*(4), 449–465. https://doi.org/10.1057/biosoc.2013.23

Leonelli, S. (2016). *Data-centric biology. A philosophical study*. University Of Chicago Press.

Leonelli, S. (2020). Learning from data journeys. In S. Leonelli & N. Tempini (Eds.), *Data journeys in the sciences* (pp. 1–24). Springer.

Levin, L., & Danesh-Meyer, H. (2010). Lost in translation. Bumps in the road between bench and bedside. *JAMA, 303*(15), 1533–1534. https://doi.org/10.1001/jama.2010.463

Levy, D., & Brink, S. (2005). *A change of heart. How the Framingham heart study helped unravel the mysteries of cardiovascular disease*. Alfred A. Knopf.

Levy, D., Splansky, G. L., Strand, N. K., Atwood, L. D., Benjamin, E. J., Blease, S., Cupples, L. A., et al. (2010). Consent for genetic research in the Framingham heart study. *American Journal of Medical Genetics Part A, 152A*(5), 1250–1256. https://doi.org/10.1002/ajmg.a.33377

Lieb, W., Strathmann, E. A., Röder, C., Jacobs, G., Gaede, K. I., Richter, G., Illig, T., & Krawczak, M. (2024). Population-based biobanking. *Genes, 15*(1). https://doi.org/10.3390/genes15010066

Lim, R. (2002). *Got Singapore. Bits and pieces from a dot in the world*. Angsana Books.

Lim, M.-K. (2010). Health care reforms in Singapore. In K. Okma & L. Crivelli (Eds.), *Six countries, six reform models: The healthcare reform experience of Israel, The Netherlands, New Zealand, Singapore, Switzerland and Taiwan* (pp. 111–136). World Scientific.

Lingle, C., & Wickman, K. (1999). Political economy. In M. Haas (Ed.), *The Singapore puzzle* (pp. 55–75). Praeger.

Lipphardt, V. (2010). Knowing Europe, Europeanizing knowledge: The making of 'homo Europaeus' in the life sciences. In M. Conway & K. K. Patel (Eds.), *Europeanization in the twentieth century: Historical approaches* (pp. 64–83). Palgrave Macmillan UK. https://doi.org/10.1057/9780230293120_4

Litton, J.-E. (2018). Launch of an infrastructure for health research: BBMRI-ERIC. *Biopreservation and Biobanking, 16*(3), 233–241. https://doi.org/10.1089/bio.2018.0027

Lorway, R., & Khan, S. (2014). Reassembling epidemiology: Mapping, monitoring and making-up people in the context of HIV prevention in India. *Social Science & Medicine, 112*, 51–62. https://doi.org/10.1016/j.socscimed.2014.04.034

Low, L. (2004). Imagining the Singapore economy in the next lap. In K. C. Ban, A. Pakir, & C. K. Tong (Eds.), *Imagining Singapore* (2nd ed., pp. 165–187). Eastern Universities Press.

Magnette, P. (2005). *Citizenship: The history of an idea*. ECPR Press.

Mamo, L., & Fishman, J. (2013). Why justice?: Introduction to the special issue on entanglements of science, ethics, and justice. *Science, Technology & Human Values, 38*(2), 159–175. https://doi.org/10.1177/0162243912473162

Marcus, G. (1995). *Technoscientific imaginaries. Conversations, profiles, and memoirs*. University of Chicago Press.

Marmot, M. (2015). *The health gap. The challenge of an unequal world.* Bloomsbury.

Marres, N. (2007). The issues deserve more credit: Pragmatist contributions to the study of public involvement in controversy. *Social Studies of Science, 37*(5), 759–780. https://doi.org/10.1177/0306312706077367

Martin, P. (2018). Genomic hope: Promise in the bioeconomy. In S. Gibbon, B. Prainsack, S. Hilgartner, & J. Lamoreaux (Eds.), *Routledge handbook of genomics, health and society* (pp. 79–89). Routledge.

Mascalzoni, D. (2015). Ethics law and governance of biobanking: A very complex normative puzzle. In D. Mascalzoni (Ed.), *Ethics, law and governance of biobanking: National, European and international approaches* (pp. 1–14). Springer Netherlands. https://doi.org/10.1007/978-94-017-9573-9_1

Mauron, A. (2008). Introduction: Biobanks, genomics, and research – A nightmare for public policy makers? In B. Elger, N. Biller-Adorno, A. Mauron, & A. Capron (Eds.), *Ethical issues in governing biobanks. Global perspectives* (pp. 1–9). Ashgate.

Mayrhofer, M., Holub, P., Wutte, A., & Litton, J.-E. (2016). BBMRI-ERIC: The novel gateway to biobanks. From humans to humans. *Bundesgesundheitsblatt, 59*(3), 379–384. https://doi.org/10.1007/s00103-015-2301-8

McGoey, L. (2015). *No such thing as a free gift. The gates foundation and the price of philanthropy*. Verso.

McGoey, L., Reiss, J., & Wahlberg, A. (2011). The global health complex. *BioSocieties, 6*(1), 1–9. https://doi.org/10.1057/biosoc.2010.45

McNeil, M., Arribas-Ayllon, M., Haran, J., Mackenzie, A., & Tutton, R. (2017). Conceptualizing imaginaries of science, technology, and society. In U. Felt, R. Fouche, C. Miller, & L. Smith-Doerr (Eds.), *The handbook of science and technology studies* (4th ed., pp. 435–464). The MIT Press.

McWhirter, R., Critchley, C., Nicol, D., Chalmers, D., Whitton, T., Otlowski, M., Burgess, M., & Dickinson, J. (2014). Community engagement for big epidemiology: Deliberative democracy as a tool. *Journal of Personalized Medicine, 4*, 459–474. https://doi.org/10.3390/jpm4040459

Mejias, U., & Couldry, N. (2019). Datafication. *Internet Policy Review. Journal on Internet Regulation, 8*(4), 1–10. https://doi.org/10.14763/2019.4.1428

Meslin, E., Blasimme, A., & Cambon-Thomsen, A. (2013). Mapping the translational science policy 'valley of death'. *Clinical and Translational Medicine, 2*(1), 14. https://doi.org/10.1186/2001-1326-2-14

Metzler, I. (2020). Imaginaries as infrastructures? The emergence of non-invasive prenatal testing in Austria. *BioSocieties, 15*(4), 601–626. https://doi.org/10.1057/s41292-019-00171-7

Metzler, I., & Åm, H. (2022). How the governance of and through digital contact tracing technologies shapes geographies of power. *Policy & Politics, 50*(2), 181–198. https://doi.org/10.1332/030557321X16420096592965

Metzler, I., Ferent, L.-M., & Felt, U. (2023). On samples, data, and their mobility in biobanking: How imagined travels help to relate samples and data. *Big Data & Society, 10*, 1–13. https://doi.org/10.1177/20539517231158635

Michael, M. (2009). Publics performing publics: Of PiGs, PiPs and politics. *Public Understanding of Science, 18*(5), 617–631. https://doi.org/10.1177/0963662508098581

Mikkelsen, R. B., Gjerris, M., Waldemar, G., & Sandøe, P. (2019). Broad consent for biobanks is best – Provided it is also deep. *BMC Medical Ethics, 20*(1), 71. https://doi.org/10.1186/s12910-019-0414-6

Miller, M. S., Gardner, T. J., Krammer, F., Aguado, L. C., Tortorella, D., Basler, C. F., & Palese, P. (2013). Neutralizing antibodies against previously encountered influenza virus strains increase over time: A longitudinal analysis. *Science Translational Medicine, 5*(198), 198ra107. https://doi.org/10.1126/scitranslmed.3006637

Misa, T., & Schot, J. (2005). Introduction: Inventing Europe: Technology and the hidden integration of Europe. *History and Technology, 21*(1), 1–19. https://doi.org/10.1080/07341510500037487

Mitchell, T. (2002). *Rule of experts: Egypt, techno-politics, and modernity*. University of California Press.

Mohapatra, B., Warrell, D., Suraweera, W., Bhatia, P., Dhingra, N., Jotkar, R., Rodriguez, P., Mishra, K., Whitaker, R., & Jha, P. (2011). Snakebite mortality in India: A nationally representative mortality survey. *PLoS Neglected Tropical Diseases, 5*(4), e1018. https://pubmed.ncbi.nlm.nih.gov/21532748/

Mol, A. (1999). Ontological politics. A word and some questions. In J. Law & J. Hassard (Eds.), *Actor network theory and after* (pp. 74–89). Blackwell.

Mol, A. (2003). *The body multiple. Ontology in medical practice.* Duke University Press.

Moreira, T. (2019). Devicing future populations: Problematizing the relationship between quantity and quality of life. *Social Studies of Science, 49*(1), 118–137. https://doi.org/10.1177/0306312719829841

Moskovko, M., Astvaldsson, A., & Hallonsten, O. (2019). Who is ERIC? The politics and jurisprudence of a governance tool for collaborative European research infrastructures. *Journal of Contemporary European Research, 15*(3), 249–268. https://doi.org/10.30950/jcer.v15i3.1028

Mouffe, C. (2011). *On the political.* Routledge.

Müller, S. (2022). Is there a civic duty to support medical AI development by sharing electronic health records? *BMC Medical Ethics, 23*(1), 134. https://doi.org/10.1186/s12910-022-00871-z

Murphy, M. (2017). *The economization of life.* Duke University Press.

Murtagh, M. J., Demir, I., Harris, J. R., & Burton, P. R. (2011). Realizing the promise of population biobanks: A new model for translation. *Human Genetics, 130*(3), 333–345. https://doi.org/10.1007/s00439-011-1036-3

Mutalib, H. (2004). Singapore's quest for a National Identity: The triumphs and trials of government policies. In K. C. Ban, A. Pakir, & C. K. Tong (Eds.), *Imagining Singapore* (2nd ed., pp. 54–80). Eastern Universities Press.

Myers, R., & O'Donnell, C. J. (1999). Genetics. In D. Levy (Ed.), *50 years of discovery. Medical milestones from the National Heart, Lung, and Blood Institute's Framingham heart study* (pp. 549–550). Center for Biomedical Communication.

Nadim, T. (2016). Data labours: How the sequence databases GenBank and EMBL-Bank make data. *Science as Culture, 25*(4), 496–519. https://doi.org/10.1080/09505431.2016.1189894

Nature. (2010). Singapore's Salad days are over. *Nature, 468*, 731. https://doi.org/10.1038/468731a

Ndambo, M. K., Reynolds, R. M., Bunn, C., Pickersgill, M., Stewart, R. C., Crampin, A. C., Nyasulu, M., et al. (2024). Can biosampling really be 'non-invasive'? An examination of the socially invasive nature of physically non-invasive biosampling in urban and rural Malawi. *Global Bioethics, 35*(1), 2398303. https://doi.org/10.1080/11287462.2024.2398303

Neher, C. (1999). The case for Singapore. In M. Haas (Ed.), *The Singapore puzzle* (pp. 39–54). Praeger.

Niewöhner, J., & Scheffer, T. (2010). Thickening comparison: On the multiple facets of comparability. In J. Niewöhner & T. Scheffer (Eds.), *Thick comparison: Reviving the ethnographic aspiration* (pp. 1–15). Brill.

Normile, D. (2007). An Asian tiger's bold experiment. *Science, 316*, 38–41. https://doi.org/10.1126/science.316.5821.38

Normile, D. (2011). Winds of change leave bioscientists scrambling. *Science, 332*, 165. https://doi.org/10.1126/science.332.6026.165

Novas, C., & Rose, N. (2000). Genetic risk and the birth of the 'somatic individual'. *Economy and Society, 29*, 485–513. https://doi.org/10.1080/030851400050174750

Nowotny, H. (2014). Engaging with the political imaginaries of science: Near misses and future targets. *Public Understanding of Science, 23*(1), 16–20. https://doi.org/10.1177/0963662513476220

O'Neil, C. (2016). *Weapons of math destruction. How big data increases inequality and threatens democracy*. Penguin Books.

Office of the Registrar General of India. (2009). *Report on causes of death in India 2001–2003*. Office of the Registrar General of India.

Office of the Registrar General of India. (2013). *Sample registration system statistical report 2011. Report No.1 of 2013*. Office of the Registrar General & Census Commissioner, India.

Ong, A. (2006a). Mutations in citizenship. *Theory, Culture & Society, 23*(2–3), 499–505. https://doi.org/10.1177/0263276406064831

Ong, A. (2006b). *Neoliberalism as exception. Mutations in citizenship and sovereignty*. Duke University Press.

Ong, A. (2013). A milieu of mutations: The pluripotency and fungibility of life in Asia. *East Asian Science, Technology, and Society: An International Journal, 7*(2), 69–85. https://doi.org/10.1215/18752160-2075241

Ong, A. (2015). Why Singapore Trumps Iceland. Gathering genes in the wild. *Journal of Cultural Economy, 8*(3), 325. https://doi.org/10.1080/17530350.2015.1009149

Ong, A., & Chen, N. (2010). *Asian biotech. Ethics and communities of fate*. Duke University Press.

Oppenheimer, G. M. (2005). Becoming the Framingham study 1947–1950. *American Journal of Public Health, 95*(4), 602–610. https://doi.org/10.2105/ajph.2003.026419

Oppenheimer, G. M. (2010). Framingham heart study: The first 20 years. *Progress in Cardiovascular Diseases, 53*(1), 55–61. https://doi.org/10.1016/j.pcad.2010.03.003

Otlowski, M. (2009). Developing an appropriate consent model for biobanks: In defence of 'broad' consent. In J. Kaye & M. Stranger (Eds.), *Principles and practice of biobank governance*. Ashgate.

Overby, C., Maloney, K., Alestock, T., Chavez, J., Berman, D., Sharaf, R., Fitzgerald, T., et al. (2015). Prioritizing approaches to engage community members and build trust in biobanks: A survey of attitudes and opinions of adults with outpatient practices at the University of Maryland. *Journal of Personalized Medicine, 5*, 264–279. https://doi.org/10.3390/jpm5030264

Owen Schaefer, G., Emanuel, E., & Wertheimer, A. (2009). The obligation to participate in biomedical research. *JAMA, 302*(1), 67–72. https://doi.org/10.1001/jama.2009.931

Pagden, A. (Ed.). (2002). *The idea of Europe. From antiquity to the European Union*. Cambridge University Press.

Palit, C. (2005). Epidemics and empire: A critique of public health policy in colonial India. In C. Palit & A. K. Dutta (Eds.), *History of medicine in India. The medical encounter* (pp. 35–47). Kalpaz Publications.

Papon, P. (2004). European scientific cooperation and research infrastructures: Past tendencies and future prospects. *Minerva, 42*(1), 61–76. https://doi.org/10.1023/B:MINE.0000017700.63978.4a

Parodi, B. (2015). Biobanks: A definition. In D. Mascalzoni (Ed.), *Ethics, law and governance of biobanking* (pp. 15–19). Springer.

Parry, B., & Greenhough, B. (2018). *Bioinformation*. Polity Press.

Parthasarathy, S. (2007). *Building genetic medicine. Breast cancer, technology, and the comparative politics of health care*. The MIT Press.

Parthasarathy, S. (2017). *Patent politics. Life forms, markets & the public*. The University of Chicago Press.

Patel, S. S. (2012). Methods and management: NIH administrators, federal oversight, and the Framingham heart study. *Bulletin of the History of Medicine, 86*(1), 94–121. https://doi.org/10.1353/bhm.2012.0017

Patel, K. (2018). *Projekt Europa. Eine Kritische Geschichte*. C.H. Beck.

Pavone, V., & Goven, J. (2017). *Bioeconomies. Life, technology, and capital in the 21st century*. Palgrave Macmillan.

Pennington, H. (2022). *COVID-19: The postgenomic pandemic*. Polity Press.

Petersen, A. (2011). *The politics of bioethics*. Routledge.

Petersen, A., & Krisjansen, I. (2015). Assembling 'the bioeconomy': Exploiting the power of the promissory life sciences. *Journal of Sociology, 51*(1), 28–46. https://doi.org/10.1177/1440783314562314

Petryna, A. (2004). Biological citizenship: The science and politics of Chernobyl-exposed populations. *Osiris, 19*, 250–265. https://doi.org/10.1086/649405

Pfister, T. (2012). *The activation of citizenship in Europe*. Cambridge University Press.

Pfotenhauer, S., & Jasanoff, S. (2017). Panacea or diagnosis? Imaginaries of innovation and the 'MIT model' in three political cultures. *Social Studies of Science, 47*(6), 783–810. https://doi.org/10.1177/0306312717706110

Pfotenhauer, S., & Juhl, J. (2017). Innovation and the political state: Beyond the myth of technologies and markets. In B. Godin & D. Vinck (Eds.), *Critical studies of innovation: Alternative approaches to the pro-innovation bias* (pp. 68–94). Edward Elgar.

Pfotenhauer, S., Juhl, J., & Aarden, E. (2019). Challenging the 'deficit model' of innovation: Framing policy issues under the innovation imperative. *Research Policy, 48*(4), 895–904. https://doi.org/10.1016/j.respol.2018.10.015

Pfotenhauer, S., Laurent, B., Papageorgiou, K., & Stilgoe, J. (2022). The politics of scaling. *Social Studies of Science, 52*(1), 3–34. https://doi.org/10.1177/03063127211048945

Phalkey, J. (2013). Introduction. Focus: Science, history, and modern India. *Isis, 104*(2), 330–336. https://doi.org/10.1086/670950

Pickering, A. (1992). From science as knowledge to science as practice. In A. Pickering (Ed.), *Science as practice and culture* (pp. 1–26). University of Chicago Press. https://doi.org/10.7208/9780226668208-002

Pickersgill, M. (2020). Pandemic sociology. *Engaging Science, Technology, and Society, 6*, 347–350. https://doi.org/10.17351/ests2020.523

Pinel, C. (2021). Renting valuable assets: Knowledge and value production in academic science. *Science, Technology & Human Values, 46*(2), 275–297. https://doi.org/10.1177/0162243920911974

Pinel, C., & Svendsen, M. N. (2021). In search of 'extra data': Making tissues flow from personal to personalised medicine. *Big Data & Society, 8*(2), 20539517211035664. https://doi.org/10.1177/20539517211035664

Pinel, C., Prainsack, B., & McKevitt, C. (2020). Caring for data: Value creation in a data-intensive research laboratory. *Social Studies of Science, 50*(2), 175–197. https://doi.org/10.1177/0306312720906567

Plows, A., & Boddington, P. (2006). Troubles with biocitizenship? *Genomics, Society and Policy, 2*(3), 115–135. https://doi.org/10.1186/1746-5354-2-3-115

Pollock, A. (2012). *Medicating race. Heart disease and durable preoccupations with difference*. Duke University Press.

Pollock, A., & Subramaniam, B. (2016). Resisting power, retooling justice: Promises of feminist postcolonial technosciences. *Science, Technology & Human Values, 41*(6), 951–966. https://doi.org/10.1177/0162243916657879

Porter, T. M. (1996). *Trust in numbers* (Reprint edition). Princeton University Press.

Prainsack, B. (2017). *Personalized medicine. Empowered patients in the 21st century?* New York University Press.

Prainsack, B. (2018). The 'we' in the 'me': Solidarity and health care in the era of personalized medicine. *Science, Technology & Human Values, 43*(1), 21–44. https://doi.org/10.1177/0162243917736139

Prasad, A. (2014a). Entangled histories and imaginative geographies of technoscientific innovations. *Science as Culture, 23*(3), 432–439. http://dx.doi.org/10.1080/09505431.2014.927629

Prasad, A. (2014b). *Imperial technoscience. Transnational histories of MRI in the United States, Britain and India*. The MIT Press.

Prasad, A. (2016). Discursive contextures of science: Euro/west-centrism and science and technology studies. *Engaging Science, Technology, and Society, 2*, 193–207. https://doi.org/10.17351/ests2016.71

Pullman, D., Etchegary, H., Gallagher, K., Hodgkinson, K., Keough, M., Morgan, D., & Street, C. (2012). Personal privacy, public benefits, and biobanks: A conjoint analysis of policy priorities and public perceptions. *Genetics in Medicine, 14*(2), 229–235. https://doi.org/10.1038/gim.0b013e31822e578f

Rabinow, P. (2005). Artificiality and enlightenment: From sociobiology to biosociality. In *Anthropologies of modernity* (pp. 179–193). Wiley. https://doi.org/10.1002/9780470775875.ch7

Rabinow, P., & Rose, N. (2006). Biopower Today. *BioSocieties, 1*, 195–217. https://doi.org/10.1017/S1745855206040014

Radin, J. (2013). Latent life: Concepts and practices of human tissue preservation in the international biological program. *Social Studies of Science, 43*(4), 484–508. https://doi.org/10.1177/0306312713476131

Radin, J. (2014). Unfolding epidemiological stories: How the WHO made frozen blood into a flexible resource for the future. *Studies in History and Philosophy of Science Part C: Studies in History and Philosophy of Biological and Biomedical Sciences, 47*, 62–73. https://doi.org/10.1016/j.shpsc.2014.05.007

Rajan, V., & Prabhakaran, D. (2012). Non-communicable diseases in India: Transitions, burden of disease and risk factors – A short story. *India Health Beat. Supporting Evidence-Based Policies and Implementation, 6*(1), 1–8.

Raman, S., & Tutton, R. (2010). Life, science, and biopower. *Science, Technology & Human Values, 35*(5), 711–734. https://doi.org/10.1177/0162243909345838

Rao, M. (2001). Eliding history. The World Bank's health policies. In D. Kumar (Ed.), *Disease and medicine in India. A historical overview* (pp. 265–275). Tulika Books.

Rao, M., Godajkar, P., Baru, R., Bisht, R., Mehrotra, R., Dasgupta, R., Reddy, S., & Bajpal, V. (2015). Draft National Health Policy 2013: A public health analysis. *Economic & Political Weekly, 50*(17), 94–101.

Reardon, J. (2013). On the emergence of science and justice. *Science, Technology & Human Values, 38*(2), 176–200. https://doi.org/10.1177/0162243912473161

Reardon, J. (2017). *The postgenomic condition. Ethics, justice & knowledge after the genome*. University of Chicago Press.

Reichel, J. (2015). EU governance for research and ethics in biobanks. In D. Mascalzoni (Ed.), *Ethics, law and governance of biobanking. National, European and international approaches* (pp. 153–185). Springer.

Reisman, D. (2009). *Social policy in an ageing society. Age and health in Singapore*. Edward Elgar.

Rennie, S. (2011). Viewing research participation as a moral obligation. In whose interests? *Hastings Center Report, 41*, 40–47. https://doi.org/10.1353/hcr.2011.0025

Reubi, D. (2018). A genealogy of epidemiological reason: Saving lives, social surveys, and global population. *BioSocieties, 13*(1), 81–102. https://doi.org/10.1057/s41292-017-0055-2

Revi, B. (2014). T.H. Marshall and his critics: Reappraising 'social citizenship' in the twenty-first century. *Citizenship Studies, 18*(3–4), 452–464. https://doi.org/10.1080/13621025.2014.905285

Rheinberger, H.-J. (1997). *Toward a history of epistemic things. Synthesizing proteins in the test tube*. Stanford University Press.

Riegman, P. H. J., Morente, M. M., Betsou, F., de Blasio, P., & Geary, P. (2008). Biobanking for better healthcare. *Molecular Oncology, 2*(3), 213–222. https://doi.org/10.1016/j.molonc.2008.07.004

Roberts, W. C. (2000). *Facts and ideas from anywhere*. Futura Publishing Company.

Roberts, C., & Tutton, R. (2018). The rise of health activism: The importance of social class to biosociality. In K. E. Happe, J. Johnson, & M. Levina (Eds.), *The politics of bodies, governance, and power* (pp. 204–221). New York University Press. https://doi.org/10.18574/nyu/9781479845194.003.0010

Rodríguez-Navarro, A., & Narin, F. (2017). European paradox or delusion – Are European science and economy outdated? *Science and Public Policy, 45*(1), 14–23. https://doi.org/10.1093/scipol/scx021

Rose, N. (2001). The politics of life itself. *Theory, Culture & Society, 18*(6), 1–30. https://doi.org/10.1177/02632760122052020

Rose, N., & Novas, C. (2005). Biological citizenship. In A. Ong & S. Collier (Eds.), *Global assemblages. Technology, politics, and ethics as anthropological problems* (pp. 439–463). Blackwell Publishing.

Rosenberg, C. (2002). The tyranny of diagnosis: Specific entities and individual experience. *The Milbank Quarterly, 80*(2), 237–260. https://doi.org/10.1111/1468-0009.t01-1-00003
Rothstein, W. (2003). *Public health and the risk factor. A history of an uneven medical revolution*. University of Rochester Press.
Rothstein, M. A. (2005). Expanding the ethical analysis of biobanks. *The Journal of Law, Medicine & Ethics, 33*(1), 89–101. https://doi.org/10.1111/j.1748-720X.2005.tb00213.x
Ruppert, E. (2011). Population objects: Interpassive subjects. *Sociology, 45*(2), 218–233. https://doi.org/10.1177/0038038510394027
Ruppert, E., & Scheel, S. (2021). *Data practices. Making up a European people*. Goldsmiths Press.
Ruppert, E., Isin, E., & Bigo, D. (2017). Data politics. *Big Data & Society, 4*, 1–7. https://doi.org/10.1177/2053951717717749
Ryan, L. (2021). European integration, the European research area and European research infrastructures. In T. Hoerber, G. Weber, & I. Cabras (Eds.), *The Routledge handbook of European integrations* (pp. 285–310). Routledge.
Saetnan, A. R., Lomell, H. M., & Hammer, S. (2011). Introduction: By the very act of counting: The mutual construction of statistics and society. In A. R. Saetnan, H. M. Lomell, & S. Hammer (Eds.), *The mutual construction of statistics and society* (pp. 1–17). Routledge.
Salter, B., Zhou, Y., Datta, S., & Salter, C. (2016). Bioinformatics and the politics of innovation in the life sciences: Science and the state in the United Kingdom, China, and India. *Science, Technology & Human Values, 41*(5), 793–826. https://doi.org/10.1177/0162243916631022
Sandor, J. (2009). From private to public? Legal concepts of the right to privacy and ownership in the regulation of biobanks. In K. Dierickx & P. Borry (Eds.), *New challenges for biobanks: Ethics, law and governance* (pp. 123–135). Intersentia.
Sangaramoorthy, T., & Benton, A. (2012). Enumeration, identity, and health. *Medical Anthropology: Cross-Cultural Studies in Health and Illness., 31*(4), 287–291. https://doi.org/10.1080/01459740.2011.638684
Sassen, S. (2000). Spatialities and temporalities of the global: Elements for a theorization. *Public Culture, 12*(1), 215–232. https://doi.org/10.1215/08992363-12-1-215
Sassen, S. (2010). *The global inside the national. A research agenda for sociology*. Sociopedia.Isa. https://saskiasassen.com/pdfs/publications/the-global-inside-the-national.pdf

Schein, E. (1996). *Strategic pragmatism. The culture of Singapore's economic development board.* The MIT Press.
Schiffman, J. (1970). Section 24. The Framingham diet study: Diet and the regulation of serum cholesterol. In *The Framingham heart study. An epidemiological investigation of cardiovascular disease.* US Department of Health, Education and Welfare, National Institutes of Health.
Schipper, F., & Schot, J. (2011). Infrastructural Europeanism, or the project of building Europe on infrastructures: An introduction. *History and Technology, 27*(3), 245–264. https://doi.org/10.1080/07341512.2011.604166
Scott, J. C. (1999). *Seeing like a state: How certain schemes to improve the human condition have failed* (New edition). Yale University Press.
Seidenberg, B. (2014). *You should share your health data: Its value outweighs the privacy risk.* Wired.
Seiler, C. (2018). Can there be a moral obligation to participate in biomedical research? *European Journal of Clinical Investigation, 48*, e12896. https://doi.org/10.1111/eci.12896
Seth, S. (2009). Putting knowledge in its place: Science, colonialism, and the postcolonial. *Postcolonial Studies, 12*(4), 373–388. https://doi.org/10.1080/13688790903350633
Shankar, K., Hakken, D., & Østerlund, C. (2017). Rethinking documents. In U. Felt, R. Fouche, C. Miller, & L. Smith-Doerr (Eds.), *The handbook of science and technology studies* (4th ed., pp. 59–85). The MIT Press.
Sheehan, M. (2011). Broad consent is informed consent. *BMJ, 343*, d6900. https://doi.org/10.1136/bmj.d6900
Shickle, D., & Griffin, M. (2009). Biobanks, networks and networks of networks. In K. Dierickx & P. Borry (Eds.), *New challenges for biobanks. Ethics, law and governance* (pp. 1–18). Intersentia.
Shim, J. (2014). *Heart-sick. The politics of risk, inequality, and heart disease.* New York University Press.
Simell, B., Törnwall, O., Hämäläinen, I., Wichmann, H.-E., Anton, G., Brennan, P., Bouvard, L., et al. (2019). Transnational access to large prospective cohorts in Europe: Current trends and unmet needs. *New Biotechnology, 49*, 98–103. https://doi.org/10.1016/j.nbt.2018.10.001
Simm, Kadri. 2010. "The making of a biobank. The case of the Estonian genome project." In Yearbook 2009 of the institute for advanced studies on science, technology and society, edited by A Bamme, Günter Getzinger, and Bernhard Wieser, 129–141. : Profil Verlag.

Singh, R. (2019). Give me a database and I will raise the nation-state. *South Asia: Journal of South Asian Studies, 42*(3), 501–518. https://doi.org/10.1080/00856401.2019.1602810

Sismondo, S. (2009). *An introduction to science and technology studies.* Wiley-Blackwell.

Sleeboom-Faulkner, M. (2009). *Human genetic biobanks in Asia. Politics of trust and scientific advancement.* Routledge.

Slota, S., & Bowker, G. (2017). How infrastructures matter. In U. Felt, R. Fouche, C. Miller, & L. Smith-Doerr (Eds.), *The handbook of science and technology studies* (4th ed., pp. 529–554). The MIT Press.

Smaglik, P. (2003). Filling biopolis Singapore. *Nature, 425*, 746–747. https://doi.org/10.1038/nj6959-746a

Smilan, L. E. (2022). Broad consent—Are we asking enough? *Ethics & Human Research, 44*(5), 22–31. https://doi.org/10.1002/eahr.500140

Sparke, M. (2017). Austerity and the embodiment of neoliberalism as ill-health: Towards a theory of biological sub-citizenship. *Social Science & Medicine, 187*, 287–295. https://doi.org/10.1016/j.socscimed.2016.12.027

Splansky, G. L., Corey, D., Yang, Q., Atwood, L. D., Cupples, L. A., Benjamin, E. J., D'Agostino, R. B., et al. (2007). The third generation cohort of the National Heart, Lung, and Blood Institute's Framingham Heart Study: Design, recruitment, and initial examination. *American Journal of Epidemiology, 165*(11), 1328–1335. https://doi.org/10.1093/aje/kwm021

SRS Collaborators of the RGI-CGHR. (2011). *Prospective study of million deaths in India: Technical document no VIII: Health care professional's manual for assigning causes of deaths based on RHIME reports.* RGI-CGHR, University of Toronto.

Star, S. L. (1999). The ethnography of infrastructure. *American Behavioral Scientist, 43*(3), 377–391. https://doi.org/10.1177/00027649921955326

Star, S. L., & Ruhleder, K. (1996). Steps toward an ecology of infrastructure: Design and access for large information spaces. *Information Systems Research, 7*(1), 111–134. https://doi.org/10.1287/isre.7.1.111

Stark, Z., Glazer, D., Hofmann, O., Rendon, A., Marshall, C. R., Ginsburg, G. S., Lunt, C., et al. (2025). A call to action to scale up research and clinical genomic data sharing. *Nature Reviews Genetics, 26*(2), 141–147. https://doi.org/10.1038/s41576-024-00776-0

Staunton, C., & de Vries, J. (2020). The governance of genomic biobank research in Africa: Reframing the regulatory tilt. *Journal of Law and the Biosciences, 7*(1), lsz018. https://doi.org/10.1093/jlb/lsz018

Stephens, N., & Dimond, R. (2015a). Closure of a human tissue biobank: Individual, institutional, and field expectations during cycles of promise and disappointment. *New Genetics and Society, 34*(4), 417–436. https://doi.org/10.1080/14636778.2015.1107469

Stephens, N., & Dimond, R. (2015b). Unexpected tissue and the biobank that closed: An exploration of value and the momentariness of bio-objectification processes. *Life Sciences, Society and Policy, 11*, 14. https://doi.org/10.1186/s40504-015-0032-0

Stilgoe, J., Lock, S. J., & Wilsdon, J. (2014). Why should we promote public engagement with science? *Public Understanding of Science, 23*(1), 4–15. https://doi.org/10.1177/0963662513518154

Stranger, M., & Kaye, J. (2009). Governing biobanks: An introduction. In J. Kaye & M. Stranger (Eds.), *Principles and practice in biobank governance* (pp. 1–15). Ashgate.

Strasser, B. J. (2012). Data-driven sciences: From wonder cabinets to electronic databases. *Data-Driven Research in the Biological and Biomedical Sciences, 43*(1), 85–87. https://doi.org/10.1016/j.shpsc.2011.10.009

Street, A. (2012). Affective infrastructure: Hospital landscapes of hope and failure. *Space and Culture, 15*(1), 44–56. https://doi.org/10.1177/1206331211426061

Stuhl, F., Franke, J., & Patel, K. (2009). *Die Erfindung Des Europäers.* Kreuzberg Museum.

Subramaniam, B., Foster, L., Harding, S., Roy, D., & TallBear, K. (2017). Feminism, Postcolonialism, Technoscience. In U. Felt, R. Fouche, C. Miller, & L. Smith-Doerr (Eds.), *The handbook of science and technology studies* (4th ed.). The MIT Press.

Sunder Rajan, K. (2006). *Biocapital. The constitution of postgenomic life*. Duke University Press.

Sunder Rajan, K. (2012). *Lively capital. Biotechnologies, ethics and governance in global markets.* Duke University Press.

Sunder Rajan, K. (2013). Questions of critique for big biology: Conjuncture, agency and the global postcolonial. *BioSocieties, 8*(4), 486–490. https://doi.org/10.1057/biosoc.2013.29

Sunder Rajan, K. (2015). Courting innovation. The constitution(s) of Indian biomedicine. In S. Hilgartner, C. Miller, & R. Hagendijk (Eds.), *Science and democracy. Making knowledge and making power in the biosciences and beyond* (pp. 56–73). Routledge.

Sunder Rajan, K. (2017). *Pharmocracy. Value, politics & knowledge in global biomedicine*. Duke University Press.
Swinbanks, D. (1999). Singapore aims to become a hot spot for life sciences. *Nature, 399*, 177. https://doi.org/10.1038/20228
Takle, M., Vedeler, J. S., Schoyen, M. A., Klette-Bohler, K., & Falch-Eriksen, A. (Eds.). (2023). *Citizenship and social exclusion at the margins of the welfare state*. Routledge.
Tamminen, S. (2015). Bio-objectifying European bodies: Standardisation of biobanks in the biobanking and biomolecular resources research infrastructure. *Life Sciences, Society and Policy, 11*(1), 13. https://doi.org/10.1186/s40504-015-0031-1
Tarkkala, H. (2019). *Reorganizing biomedical research. Biobanks as conditions of possibility for personalized medicine*. University of Helsinki. https://helda.helsinki.fi/server/api/core/bitstreams/77ef4aea-e427-475a-8669-78056e529c9c/content
Tarkkala, H., & Tupasela, A. (2018). Shortcut to success? Negotiating genetic uniqueness in global biomedicine. *Social Studies of Science, 48*(5), 740–761. https://doi.org/10.1177/0306312718801165
Taussig, K. S., Hoeyer, K., & Helmreich, S. (2013). The anthropology of potentiality in biomedicine. *Current Anthropology, 54*(S7), S3–S14. https://doi.org/10.1086/671401
Thacker, E. (2005). *The global genome. Biotechnology, politics, and culture*. The MIT Press.
Thompson, C. (2010). Asian regeneration? Nationalism and internationalism in stem cell research in South Korea and Singapore. In A. Ong & N. Chen (Eds.), *Asian biotech. Ethics and communities of fate* (pp. 95–117). Duke University Press.
Thorpe, C., & Gregory, J. (2010). Producing the post-Fordist public: The political economy of public engagement with science. *Science as Culture, 19*(3), 273–301. https://doi.org/10.1080/09505430903194504
Timmermans, S., & Epstein, S. (2010). A world of standards but not a standard world: Toward a sociology of standards and standardization. *Annual Review of Sociology, 36*, 69–89. https://doi.org/10.1146/annurev.soc.012809.102629
Tindana, P., Yakubu, A., Staunton, C., Matimba, A., Littler, K., Madden, E., Munung, N. S., de Vries, J., & as members of the H3Africa Consortium. (2019). Engaging research ethics committees to develop an ethics and governance framework for best practices in genomic research and biobanking in Africa: The H3Africa model. *BMC Medical Ethics, 20*(1), 69. https://doi.org/10.1186/s12910-019-0398-2

Trischler, H., & Kohlrausch, M. (2014). *Building Europe on expertise: Innovators, organizers, networkers*. Palgrave Macmillan.

Trivedi, B. (2008). Betting the bank. *Nature, 452*(April 24), 926–929. https://doi.org/10.1038/452926a

Trocki, C. (2009). *Singapore. Wealth, power, and the culture of control*. Routledge.

Tupasela, A. (2006). Locating tissue collections in tissue economies-deriving value from biomedical research. *New Genetics and Society, 25*(1), 33–49. https://doi.org/10.1080/14636770600603469

Tupasela, A. (2017a). Data-sharing politics and the logics of competition in biobanking. In V. Pavone & J. Goven (Eds.), *Bioeconomies. Life, technology, and capital in the 21st century* (pp. 187–206). Palgrave Macmillan.

Tupasela, A. (2017b). Populations as brands in medical research: Placing genes on the global genetic atlas. *BioSocieties, 12*(1), 47–65. https://doi.org/10.1057/s41292-016-0029-9

Tupasela, A. (2021). Data hugging in European biobank networks. *Science as Culture, 30*(4), 513–534. https://doi.org/10.1080/09505431.2021.1949274

Tupasela, A., Snell, K., & Cañada, J. (2015). Constructing populations in biobanking. *Life Sciences, Society and Policy, 11*(5), 1–18. https://doi.org/10.1186/s40504-015-0024-0

Tupasela, A., Snell, K., & Tarkkala, H. (2020). The Nordic data imaginary. *Big Data & Society, 7*. https://doi.org/10.1177/2053951720907107

Turner, A., Dallaire-Fortier, C., & Murtagh, M. (2013). Biobank economics and the 'commercialization problem'. *Spontaneous Generations: A Journal for the History and Philosophy of Science, 7*(1), 69–80. http://dx.doi.org/10.4245/sponge.v7i1.19555

Tutton, R. (2007). Constructing participation in genetic databases. Citizenship, governance, and ambivalence. *Science, Technology & Human Values, 32*(2), 172–195. https://doi.org/10.1177/0162243906296853

Tutton, R. (2010). Biobanking: Social, political and ethical aspects. In *Encyclopedia of life sciences*. Wiley. https://doi.org/10.1002/9780470015902.a0022083

Van der Laan, A., & Boenink, M. (2015). Beyond bench and bedside: Disentangling the concept of translational research. *Health Care Analysis, 23*(1), 32–49. https://doi.org/10.1007/s10728-012-0236-x

Van Lente, H. (2000). Forceful futures: From promise to requirement. In N. Brown, B. Rappert, & A. Webster (Eds.), *Contested futures. A sociology of prospective techno-science* (pp. 43–64). Ashgate.

Végvári, Á., Welinder, C., Lindberg, H., Fehniger, T. E., & Marko-Varga, G. (2011). Biobank resources for future patient care: Developments, principles and concepts. *Journal of Clinical Bioinformatics, 1*(1), 24. https://doi.org/10.1186/2043-9113-1-24

Vermeulen, N., Parker, J., & Penders, B. (2013). Understanding life together: A brief history of collaboration in biology. *Endeavour, 37*(3), 162–171. https://doi.org/10.1016/j.endeavour.2013.03.001

Versluis, E. (2007). Even rules, uneven practices: Opening the 'black box' of EU Law in action. *West European Politics, 30*(1), 50–67. https://doi.org/10.1080/01402380601019647

Vignola-Gagne, E., & Biegelbauer, P. (2013). Translational research. In E. Carayannis (Ed.), *Encyclopedia of creativity, invention, innovation and entrepreneurship* (pp. 1834–1843). Springer.

Villadsen, K., & Wahlberg, A. (2015). The government of life: Managing populations, health, and scarcity. *Economy and Society, 44*(2), 1–17. https://doi.org/10.1080/03085147.2014.983831

Vimal, M., Devi, W. P., & McGonigle, I. (2023). Generational medicine in Singapore: A National Biobank for a greying nation. *East Asian Science, Technology and Society: An International Journal, 17*(1), 71–87. https://doi.org/10.1080/18752160.2021.1925388

Visvanathan, S. (2002). The future of science studies. *Futures, 34*(1), 91–101. https://doi.org/10.1016/S0016-3287(01)00037-4

Visvanathan, S. (2005). Knowledge, justice and democracy. In M. Leach, I. Scoones, & B. Wynne (Eds.), *Science and citizens. Globalization and the challenges of engagement* (pp. 83–94). Zed Books.

Vogel, G. (2012). How do you count the dead? *Science, 336*, 1372–1374. https://doi.org/10.1126/science.336.6087.1372

Von Hirschhausen, A., & Patel, K. (2010). Europeanization in history: An introduction. In M. Conway & K. Patel (Eds.), *Europeanization in the twentieth century. Historical approaches* (pp. 1–18). Palgrave Macmillan.

Vuorio, E. (2017). Networking biobanks throughout Europe: The development of BBMRI-ERIC. In P. Hainaut, P. Vaught, K. Zatloukal, & M. Pasterk (Eds.), *Biobanking of human biospecimens. Principles and practice* (pp. 137–153). Springer.

Wahlberg, A. (2022). Assemblage ethnography: Configurations across scales, sites, and practices. In M. H. Bruun, A. Wahlberg, R. Douglas-Jones, C. Hasse, K. Hoeyer, D. B. Kristensen, & B. R. Winthereik (Eds.), *The Palgrave handbook of the anthropology of technology* (pp. 125–144). Palgrave Macmillan.

Wahlberg, A., & Rose, N. (2015). The governmentalization of living: Calculating global health. *Economy and Society, 44*(1), 60–90. https://doi.org/10.1080/03085147.2014.983830

Waldby, C. (2009a). Biobanking in Singapore: Post-developmental state, experimental population. *New Genetics and Society, 28*(3), 253–265. https://doi.org/10.1080/14636770903151943

Waldby, C. (2009b). Singapore biopolis: Bare life in the city-state. *East Asian Science, Technology, and Society: An International Journal, 3*, 367–383. https://doi.org/10.1007/s12280-009-9089-2

Waldby, C. (2012). Medicine: The ethics of care, the subject of experiment. *Body & Society, 18*(3–4), 179–192. https://doi.org/10.1177/1357034X12451778

Waldby, C., & Mitchell, R. (2006). *Tissue economies. Blood, organs, and cell lines in late capitalism*. Duke University Press.

Ward, J. S., & Barker, A. (2013). *Undefined by data: A survey of big data definitions*. https://arxiv.org/abs/1309.5821

Watson, P., Nussbeck, S., Carter, C., O'Donoghue, S., Cheah, S., Matzke, L., Barnes, R., et al. (2014). A framework for biobank sustainability. *Biopreservation and Biobanking, 12*(1), 60–68. https://doi.org/10.1089/bio.2013.0064

Watson, O. J., Barnsley, G., Toor, J., Hogan, A. B., Winskill, P., & Ghani, A. C. (2022). Global impact of the first year of COVID-19 vaccination: A mathematical modelling study. *The Lancet Infectious Diseases, 22*(9), 1293–1302. https://doi.org/10.1016/S1473-3099(22)00320-6

Widdows, H., & Cordell, S. (2011). The ethics of biobanking: Key issues and controversies. *Health Care Analysis, 19*(3), 207–219. https://doi.org/10.1007/s10728-011-0184-x

Widdows, H., & Mullen, C. (2009). *The governance of genetic information. Who decides?* Cambridge University Press.

Wiertz, S., & Boldt, J. (2022). Evaluating models of consent in changing Health Research environments. *Medicine, Health Care and Philosophy, 25*(2), 269–280. https://doi.org/10.1007/s11019-022-10074-3

Wilkinson, M. D., Dumontier, M., Aalbersberg, I. J. J., Appleton, G., Axton, M., Baak, A., Blomberg, N., et al. (2016). The FAIR guiding principles for scientific data management and stewardship. *Scientific Data, 3*(1), 160018. https://doi.org/10.1038/sdata.2016.18

Will, C. M., & Bendelow, G. (2020). Processing the pandemic. *Sociology of Health & Illness, 42*(8), 1–3. https://doi.org/10.1111/1467-9566.13222

Wimmer, A., & Schiller, N. G. (2003). Methodological nationalism, the social sciences, and the study of migration: An essay in historical epistemology. *International Migration Review, 37*(3), 576–610. https://doi.org/10.1111/j.1747-7379.2003.tb00151.x

Winickoff, D. (2006). Genome and nation: Iceland's health sector database and its legacy. *Innovations, 1*(2), 80–105. https://doi.org/10.1162/itgg.2006.1.2.80

Winner, L. (1986). *The whale and the reactor. A search for limits in an age of high technology*. The University of Chicago Press.

Wohlfarth, A. (2020). Renegotiating social citizenship – Democracy in welfare service states. *Social Work & Society, 18*(1), 1–10. https://www.socwork.net/sws/article/view/613

Wong, J. (2011). *Betting on biotech. Innovation and the limits of Asia's developmental state*. Cornell University Press.

Woolf, S. (2008). The meaning of translational research and why it matters. *JAMA, 299*(2), 211–213. https://doi.org/10.1001/jama.2007.26

World Health Organization. (2010). Save lives by counting the dead. Interview with Prabhat Jha. *Bulletin of the World Health Organization, 88*(3), 171.

Wynne, B. (2006). Public engagement as a means of restoring trust in science – Hitting the notes, but missing the music? *Community Genetics, 9*, 211–220. https://doi.org/10.1159/000092659

Wynne, B. (2007). Public participation in science and technology: Performing and obscuring a political-conceptual category mistake. *East Asian Science, Technology, and Society: An International Journal., 1*(1), 99–110. https://doi.org/10.1007/s12280-007-9004-7

Yao, S. (2007). *Singapore. The state and the culture of excess*. Routledge.

Yates-Doerr, E. (2020). Reworking the social determinants of health: Responding to material-semiotic indeterminacy in public health interventions. *Medical Anthropology Quarterly, 34*(4), 378–397. https://doi.org/10.1111/maq.12586

Yew, L. (2011). A brief history of the hub: Navigating between 'global' and 'Asian' in Singapore's knowledge economy discourse. In D. Heng & S. M. K. Aljunied (Eds.), *Singapore in global history* (pp. 269–290). Amsterdam University Press.

Yuille, M., van Ommen, G. J., Brechot, C., Cambon-Thomsen, A., Dagher, G., Landegren, U., Litton, J. E., et al. (2007). Biobanking for Europe. *Briefings in Bioinformatics, 9*(1), 14–24. https://doi.org/10.1093/bib/bbm050

Zatloukal, K., Vuorio, E., & Dagher, G. (2012). BBMRI business plan, V21.1, 3.12.2012. http://www.meduni07.edis.at/files/bbmri_business_plan_v21.1_cover.pdf

Zielhuis, G. A. (2012). Biobanking for epidemiology. *Public Health, 126*(3), 214–216. https://doi.org/10.1016/j.puhe.2011.12.007

Index

E. Aarden, *Producing Citizenship in Medical Research Collections*, Health, Technology and Society, https://doi.org/10.1007/978-981-95-1707-7

T

U

V

FSC
www.fsc.org
MIX
Papier | Fördert
gute Waldnutzung
FSC® C083411

Kolibri 360 GmbH
Ferdinand-Jühlke-Straße 7
99095 Erfurt, Deutschland
produktsicherheit@kolibri360.de